America
Off The Wall

The West Coast

Travel Books from Wiley

DO'S AND TABOOS AROUND THE WORLD
Edited by Roger E. Axtell

PASSPORT TO EUROPE'S SMALL HOTELS AND INNS–27th Edition
Beverly Beyer

FESTIVALS U.S.A.
Kathleen Hill

THE BED & BREAKFAST DIRECTORY
Barbara Notarius

EUROPE OFF THE WALL
Anneli S. Rufus & Kristan Lawson

America
Off The Wall

The West Coast
A Guide to Unusual Sights

Kristan Lawson
and
Anneli S. Rufus

WILEY
John Wiley & Sons, Inc.
New York • Chichester • Brisbane
Toronto • Singapore

Publisher: Stephen Kippur
Editor: Katherine Schowalter
Managing Editor: Ruth Greif
Editing, Design, Typesetting, and Production:
  Northeastern Graphic Services, Inc.

Illustrations by Anneli S. Rufus
Maps by Kristan Lawson

This publication is designed to provide accurate and authoritative information in regard to the subject matter covered. It is sold with the understanding that the publisher is not engaged in rendering professional services. Due to the ever-changing marketplace, we suggest that you contact the addresses given to verify information.

Library of Congess Cataloging-in-Publication Data

Lawson, Kristan.
   America off the wall: the West Coast: a guide to unusual sights
   /Kristan Lawson, Anneli Rufus.
        p.   cm.
   ISBN 0-471-62269-9
   1. Pacific States--Description and travel--1981---Guide-books.
I. Rufus, Anneli S.   II. Title.
F851.L434   1989
917.9'0433--dc19   88-26896
                                                      CIP

Printed in the United States of America
89 90 10 9 8 7 6 5 4 3 2 1

Contents

ACKNOWLEDGMENTS

The authors would like to thank the following people:

Susie Lee, Donald Frew, Laura Hagar, Deborah Martin, Howard Morrill, David Rufus, Marcia Rufus, Ina Lawson, H.R. Lawson, Michael Gene Anderson, Charles Margolis, Sylvia Fuerstenberg, Richard Senate, and Joni Fassett.

HOW TO
USE THIS GUIDE

This Guide is divided into nine chapters, each of which is based on a geographical region. The cities within each region appear in alphabetical order. The first six chapters are devoted to regions of California; the other chapters are devoted to entire states.

The bottoms of the pages also serve as a quick alphabetical index to *America Off The Wall: The West Coast*: the left-hand pages list the region or state; the right-hand pages list the cities that appear on each page.

In addition to a complete index of cities at the back of the book, you'll also find the following special indexes:

Buildings Shaped Like Things

Eccentric Art

Fairytale Parks

Food Festivals

Ghost Towns

Mystery Spots

Renaissance and Medieval Faires

Sand Castle Contests

Slug Festivals

CALIFORNIA

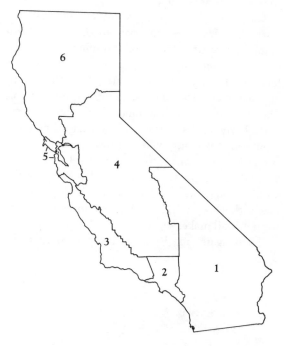

Regions:
1. San Diego and the South
2. Los Angeles and Orange County
3. The Central Coast
4. The Central Valley and the Gold Country
5. The San Francisco Bay Area
6. The North

California is overdue for a promotion. Other, less impressive spots, such as Uruguay and Bulgaria, are full-fledged nations. Australia and Antarctica, neither of which are overly exciting, both rank as continents. And yet California is still nothing more than a lowly state, no more politically advanced than Delaware, Iowa or South Carolina. Studies have shown that if California were an independent country, it would be the ninth wealthiest nation on earth; it would be the world's largest exporter of fruits and vegetables; it would control the international markets for computers, blue jeans, and made-for-TV movies; and it would have more off-the-wall sights per capita than any other country.

California didn't get this way by accident. For starters, it was blessed with incomparable geographic diversity. Its natural resources attracted everyone from wealthy entrepreneurs to menial laborers. Then, most importantly, came the visionary madmen, the outcasts, the eccentrics, all drawn inexorably to the land where dreams come true. Early in its history, California earned the reputation of being wild, innovative, and weird. It's still wild, innovative, and weird. Especially weird. Crazy attractions come thick and fast in the Golden State. There are so many off-the-wall places that we've divided the state into six regions so that it all makes sense.

Then again, maybe it isn't supposed to make sense.

SAN DIEGO AND THE SOUTH

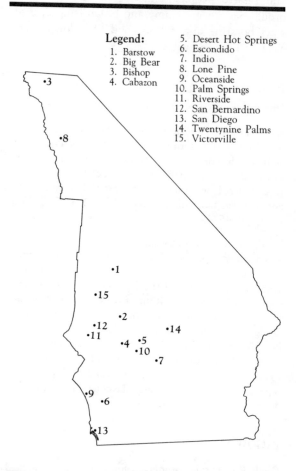

Legend:
1. Barstow
2. Big Bear
3. Bishop
4. Cabazon
5. Desert Hot Springs
6. Escondido
7. Indio
8. Lone Pine
9. Oceanside
10. Palm Springs
11. Riverside
12. San Bernardino
13. San Diego
14. Twentynine Palms
15. Victorville

Don't go thinking that the beach is all there is to Southern California. In her infinite wisdom, Nature placed there, between sea, forest, and mountains, a desert. And a perfect desert it is: lots of sand and not much water, dotted with the hard-baked houses of wily desert rats.

Every child who has grown up in Southern California cherishes a strange desert tale or two: travelers dying of thirst in their cars, a lost Spanish mission filled with gold, sailing ships emerging ghostlike from the sand, Jesus Christ hitchhiking on Route 66.

California thrives on legends of bizarre places and bizarre people. This region does the state proud. San Diego, balmy and beach-fringed, is always boasting about "the good life" down there. Yeah? So how do you explain Death Valley?

BALLARAT
(45 miles north of Ridgecrest)

Ghost Town: From Ridgecrest go east on Highway 178 for 13 miles, then turn north to the town of Trona; continue north past Trona for 18 miles until you come to a dirt road on your right. Drive east on this dirt road for three miles. It will take you straight to Ballarat. Visible anytime. For more information, Call (619) 375-7125 or (619) 375-4524.

Only three of Ballarat's tumbledown buildings have survived the ravages of wind, time, and vandals. Once a major supply center for miners, Ballarat was abandoned years ago when most of the local prospectors wandered away to richer pickings. Ruins, foundations, and the outlines of once-crowded streets punctuate the barren desert landscape. A mile north of Ballarat, a different road branches to the east; it once led to Panamint City, another ghost town of shacks and mining buildings. The road was washed out in 1984 and will probably never be repaired. A rugged eight-mile hike deters all but the most determined ghost-town fiends.

BIG BEAR

Duck Race: the Saturday before Labor Day, noon–4 P.M. Maggie's Place Bar and Grill, 39904 Big Bear Boulevard (at Edgemore), in the Boulder Bay area. For more information, call (714) 866-2381.

They're off and waddling! White ducks jostle each other as they race along a 30-foot "speedway" set up in Maggie's parking lot. You say you don't like naked ducks? At the *après*-race Duck Costume Parade, prizes are awarded to the best-dressed quackers. A recent winner was a dead ringer for Dolly Parton.

Sugarloaf Cordwood Company: 42193 Big Bear Boulevard. Open Sunday–Friday, 9 A.M.–5 P.M.; Saturday, 9 A.M.–7 P.M. Phone: (714) 866-2220.

Whether or not your foyer needs a 16-foot carved wood bear, the gigantic wares on display here merit a look. The company's owner discovered chainsaw carving up north in the California redwoods, and he brought the craft down south. Towering Indians, eagles, pirates, and other unsubtle images rear their wooden heads in the one-acre display yard.

BISHOP

Mule Days: on Memorial Day weekend, Thursday–Sunday. Bishop Fairgrounds, at Main Street (Highway 395) and Sierra Street, north side of town. Shows and events happen at various times throughout the festival. Admission to each show, $7; children under 13, $2. For more information and reservations, call (619) 873-8405.

Mule Days' motto is "anything a good horse can do, a mule can do better." They mean it, too. Competitions include mule jumping, mule racing, mule chariot racing, and the whole litany of standard rodeo events, all done with mules instead of horses. Saturday's 10 A.M. Mule Parade is the longest nonmotorized parade in the country. The chaotic highlights each year are the Mule Team Packing Scrambles, in which scores of mules, cattle, horses, and mule-loving cowboys (packers) are released into the arena simultaneously. The packers are expected to retrieve their own mules from the madness. Mule owners the world over descend on Bishop this weekend to buy, sell, and show off their prized mules, so be forewarned: Every hotel for miles around is booked months in advance.

Wild West Bed Races: during the Wild West Rodeo, on Labor Day weekend. Races on Main Street, Saturday, starting at 9:30 A.M.; finals at the Bishop Fairgrounds (Main and Sierra Streets) at noon. For more information, call (619) 873-8405.

Get ready for some high-speed snoozing as Bishop's finest athletes push theme-decorated beds down Bishop's main drag. Awards go not only to the fastest bed but also to the slowest bed, the funniest bed, and the best cheaters.

BORREGO SPRINGS
(75 miles northeast of San Diego)

Peg Leg Liars' Contest: the Saturday nearest April 1 (but never on Easter Weekend), starting at dusk (around 7 P.M.). At Peg Leg Smith Monument, intersection of Henderson Canyon Road and S22, inside Anza-Borrego State Park, eight miles east of town. For more information, call (619) 767-5311.

We're not sure who's the real star here: Peg Leg Smith, legendary 1850s desert rat, prospector, and teller of tall tales...or Harry Oliver, 1930s Hollywood movie producer, Peg Leg fan and originator of the contest. April 1 is Oliver's birthday. The liars eat a cake in his honor, but the shaggy-dog yarns they spin by the campfire are pure Peg Leg. A recent winner told a tale of huntin' fer gold one bleak desert winter, gettin' caught in a snowstorm, and finally slicing open his faithful horse in a last-ditch effort to warm himself. And damn if he didn't find a fortune in gold inside the horse's intestines. Whaddya mean, ya don't believe it?

CABAZON
(14 miles northwest of Palm Springs)

Dinosaurs at the Wheel Inn: 5900 Main Street. Take the Main Street off-ramp from Highway 10. Open Wednesday–Sunday, 10 A.M.–6 P.M., but visible from the outside anytime. Admission to museum: 50¢; children, 25¢. Phone: (714) 849-8309.

We spent the '60s watching "Gilligan's Island." Claude Bell, owner of the Wheel Inn, spent the '60s constructing a giant green brontosaurus next to his café. Giant brontosaurus? Isn't that redundant? Nope. Bell's bronto is *bigger than life-size*. The dinosaur is hollow: you can climb inside and explore a museum of guns, coins, and old things. Also here is a gray Tyrannosaurus rex, just completed five years ago. Sorry, folks, the Tyrannosaurus' bowels are strictly off-limits. And yup, these are the same dinosaurs you loved in *Pee Wee's Big Adventure*.

CALICO
(Ten miles east of Barstow)

Calico Hullabaloo World Tobacco Spitting Championships: the Sunday before Easter (Palm Sunday), late March or early April. Spitting starts at noon, next to the Confectionery. From Barstow, go east for nine miles on Highway 15, then turn north on the Calico turnoff for about one mile. Admission: $3.50. Phone: (619) 254-2122.

This contest might be disgusting, but at least it's authentic. Much of what goes on at Calico, Knott's Berry Farm's simulated ghost town in the desert, is prettified for "family-oriented" tourists. But this event is down and dirty, the way things really were. The furthest-flung wad thus far, listed in the *Guinness Book of World Records*, flew 47 feet. Spits are judged on accuracy and distance, and anybody can compete. Start exercisin' those lips today. *Ptooi!*

CARLSBAD

Memorabilia, Ltd.: 7624 El Camino Real (at La Costa Avenue), in a shopping center just north of the La Costa Hotel and Spa. Open Monday–Saturday, 10 A.M.–5 P.M. Admission: free. Phone: (619) 436-2321.

From Ringo Starr to Richard Nixon, the gang's all here. At least, their autographs are here. Framed with taste and wit, personal letters, hastily scrawled notes, and other documents fill this cozy museum/shop. The owner is especially proud of an almost-complete set of U.S. presidents' signatures.

CERRO GORDO
(21 miles east of Lone Pine)

Ghost Town: From Lone Pine, go south on Highway 395 for one-half mile; turn southeast on Highway 136 around Owens Lake Bed for 13 miles to Keeler. From Keeler, a winding dirt road branches to the east and reaches Cerro Gordo after 7½ miles. Make sure your car is in good condition: The road gains 5,000 feet in elevation between Keeler and Cerro Gordo. Always visible. Admission: free, but donations for the restoration project are welcomed. Phone: (619) 876-4154 or (619) 876-5871.

In 1871, Cerro Gordo was the wealthiest city in the United States. Silver production matched that of Nevada's legendary Comstock Lode at Virginia City. Money from Cerro Gordo helped to build Los Angeles, and water diverted from nearby Owens Lake filled L.A.'s reservoirs. But the lake dried up, the silver ran out, and now Cerro Gordo is a ghost town. In fact, it's one of the best-preserved ghost towns in the country. Twenty-five buildings—from outhouses to hotels—still stand, most in remarkably good condition. The whole townsite is now privately owned, and the owners welcome visitors as they slowly restore the once-thriving city. Weather here can be harsh in summer and winter, so come prepared.

COACHELLA
(Four miles southeast of Indio)

Covalda Date Shop: 51392 Highway 86 (at 6th Street). Open daily, 8 A.M.–4:30 P.M. Admission: free. Phone: (619) 398-3551.

Founded in 1919, this was the first soft-date packing facility in the whole valley. Today you can take a self-guided tour of the sorting area and the candy kitchen. On the walls are photos of the local date industry's history. Pick up a map here that will guide you to the Covalda Ranch, where the palms are. This spot is unusual in that it has never been sprayed with insecticides, so it's a natural haven for birds.

DEL MAR

Frog Jumping Jamboree: the last Saturday in April, 9 A.M.–4 P.M. Del Mar Fairgrounds, just north of downtown. Main entrance is on Jimmy Durante Boulevard. Frog rental: $2; children, $1. For more information, call (619) 755-4844.

Baseball-sized frogs are borrowed for the day from a local laboratory. ("What?" squeak the frogs. "No electrodes today?") The 35-year tradition, based on Mark Twain's short story, is officially sanctioned by the mayor of Angels Camp, original home of frog-jumping contests. After competing in the "frog-launching area," many of the jumpers enter the "best-dressed frog" contest. Yes, you'll see more than your fair share of frogs dressed as princes. Frog-calling and frog-kissing contests keep the festival jumpin'.

DESERT HOT SPRINGS

Cabot's Old Indian Pueblo Museum: 67616 East Desert View Avenue (at Miracle Hill Road). Open September–June, Wednesday–Monday, 9:30 A.M.–4:30 P.M.; July–August, Friday–Monday, 10 A.M.–4 P.M. Admission: $2; seniors, $1.50; children, $1. Phone: (619) 329-7610.

Working without a blueprint, eccentric world traveler Cabot Yerxa built his house on the empty desert in 1941: a four-story, 35-room Hopi-style warren, with protruding roof beams and walls two feet thick. Yerxa built the house virtually alone, with found materials. He moved in, never quite finished construction, and died in the kitchen. After years of neglect, the pueblo has been reopened as a museum. You can explore the rooms, inspect Yerxa's collection of Indian artifacts and learn more about this man who lived just about everywhere and spoke 21 languages, including 14 Indian dialects.

Kingdom of the Dolls: 66071 Pierson Boulevard, between West Drive and Cactus Drive. Open in winter, Tuesday–Sunday, noon–5 P.M.; in summer, by appointment only. Admission: $2.50; children 75¢. Phone: (619) 329-5137.

No, it's not a scary movie about Chatty Cathies invading a town. It's an amazing array of historical dioramas, peopled by unintimidating little plastic dolls. One woman built the whole kingdom. As her hobby turned into a lifestyle, Betty Hamilton carefully researched world history, sewed authentic clothes for the dolls, and built elaborate scenarios around them. She used mostly scraps and leftovers to build her castles, carriages, and other backdrops: egg cartons, plastic curlers, bits of carpet...and she used them so cleverly that you'll feel sheepish ever throwing anything away. Twenty-four years on the project have yielded the Colosseum, a disco, and dozens more.

EL CAJON

Unarius Academy of Science: 145 South Magnolia Avenue, at Douglas Avenue, downtown. Open Monday–Saturday, 10 A.M.–9 P.M.; Sunday, noon–7 P.M. Admission: free. Phone: (619) 447-4170.

Ruth Norman, leader of Unarius, is no ordinary woman. She's the Archangel Uriel, here from another planet to raise our spiritual level. Not only that, but in the year

2001 a spaceship from the planet Myton will bring a thousand aliens to Earth to usher in the Age of Logic. Moreover, you deserve every bad thing that happens to you, because you screwed up in a previous life. Whether or not you're ready for Unarius, Unarius is ready for you. Everyone's invited to stop in at their World Headquarters to browse through the unique library (how about a copy of *Satan Is Now a Light Bearer?*). Gawk at indecipherable exhibits about Pythagoras and the Planet Brundage, and admire Ruth Norman's multicolored metallic cape. On occasional Sundays, Unarius students channel paintings from spirit guides.

ENCINITAS
(25 miles north of San Diego, on the coast)

Surfing Memorabilia Collection: at George's Restaurant, 641 Highway 101 (aka 1st Street), at E Street. (Look for the big wave mural.) Open daily, 7 A.M.–2 A.M. Admission: free. Phone: (619) 942-9549.

For years, the owner of this coffee shop offered a free breakfast to anyone who would donate a framed picture of him- or herself on a surfboard. Meanwhile she started amassing a collection of surf artifacts: almost-ancient surfboards (including some "planks" from Hawaii); a jacket belonging to one of the Surfaris; a 50-year-old tiki, former "sentinel" of nearby Windansea Beach.... In fact, the collection's so big that the owner is trying to find a new location for it. But for now you've gotta take your java along with your Jan and Dean.

ESCONDIDO
(28 miles north of San Diego)

Lawrence Welk Museum: in the Lawrence Welk Resort Village, seven miles north of town, off Highway 15. Museum is in the second building to the right as you enter the resort. Open Sunday, 10 A.M.–1 P.M.; Monday, 10 A.M.–5 P.M. Tuesday–Friday, 10 A.M.–1 P.M. and 4:15–8:30 P.M. (but closing times vary, to coordinate with show times at the Lawrence Welk Village Theater). Admission: free. Phone: (619) 749-3448.

(We *refuse* to start this entry with "A-one and a-two." We absolutely will not do it.) What you'll see here are props and instruments that were used on Welk's TV show, as well as pictures and other relics enshrining Welk and his family. Don't miss the world's largest champagne glass. It's bigger than you are, and filled with bubbly. Bubbly water, that is.

HELENDALE
(15 miles north of Victorville)

Strippers' Hall of Fame: 29053 Wild Road. Take National Trails Highway north from Highway 15 at Victorville and go 15 miles to the Helendale Market; turn left and go two miles until you come to two artificial waterfalls. Turn right there on Helendale Road. After one mile you reach Wild Road; turn right and stay on the asphalt road for one mile until you see the unmistakable iron gate; drive through the gate and you're there. Open by appointment only. Admission: $10. Phone: (619) 243-5261 or (619) 948-1153.

Stripping, says curator Jennie Lee, is becoming a thing of the past. In her own haphazard way she's out to preserve it. Jennie was once a big star in the burlesque world—and we mean *big*—but her days as "Miss 44 and Plenty More" and "The Bazoom Girl" are long gone. The Strippers' Hall of Fame is really nothing more than Jennie's cluttered home: Memorabilia from her career is strewn everywhere. Pictures of chesty naked ladies cover the walls. A heart-shaped pink couch—once used as a prop in a Jayne Mansfield movie—lies half hidden under a pile of old newspapers. Jennie blithely hands each visitor vintage booklets such as "Intimate Glimpses of Miss 44 and Plenty More," proving once and for all that her stage name was no exaggeration.

INDIO

Jensen's Date and Citrus Gardens: 80653 Highway 111, between Jefferson and Madison Streets. Open daily, 9 A.M.–5 P.M. Admission: free. Phone: (619) 347-3897.

Wander around one full acre of flourishing desert garden, wherein grow flowers, cacti, and lots of dates.

National Date Festival: ten days during mid-February, surrounding Presidents' Day weekend. Camel and ostrich racing every afternoon. Riverside County Fairgrounds, Highway 111, between Arabia and Oasis Streets, just west of Highway 86 in south-central Indio. Admission to the festival: $4; children 5–11, $2; children under 5, free. Admission to the races: $1. For current dates and more information, call (619) 342-8247.

Even Arabia itself isn't *this* much fun: Bedouin tents, camel races, pashas in satin pants, date-flavored ice cream and milkshakes, daily performances of *Scheherazade*, and a

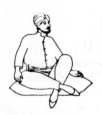

Kismet-like midway basking in the desert sun like a shimmering mirage. Is Indio a member of OPEC? Not exactly, but it is the date-growing center of the Western hemisphere. Indio's massive date crop is just an excuse for locals to turn the fairgrounds into a Middle Eastern fantasyland. Thrill seekers head straight for the comical camel and ostrich races to watch hapless jockeys struggle futilely to guide their steeds.

Shields Date Garden: 80225 Highway 111, just past Jefferson Street. Open daily, 8 A.M.–6 P.M. Admission: free. Phone: (619) 347-0996.

Late winter and early spring are the best times to visit this thriving date-o-rama. Stroll among the tall date palms, the citrus trees, and rose gardens; sample a frosty date shake. If you can handle biology, watch Shields' now-famous film *The Sex Life of a Date*.

JACUMBA
(75 miles east of San Diego)

Desert View Tower: From Jacumba, go about four miles east to Highway 8, then continue about three miles northeast on Highway 8 to the In-Ko-Pah turnoff, just before where the highway splits. Signs from the turnoff direct you one mile north to the tower, on the west side of the highway. Open daily, 8:30 A.M.–5 P.M. Admission: $1; children, 50¢. Viewing the carvings is free. Phone: (619) 766-4612.

Desert View Tower, a five-story building in the middle of nowhere, contains a museum of pioneer and Indian relics and has a lookout platform from which, on clear days, you can see over 100 miles. But that's not what you came here to see. South of the tower, on the other side of the parking lot, are boulders carved into fantastic animal shapes, strewn across the desert floor. In the 1930s a man named Ratcliffe, convalescing in the desert nearby, was inspired by the unusual forms of the desert rocks and decided to give nature a little help. He spent five years carving idiosyncratic faces, animals, and skulls out of the rocks. One lizard, basking in the sun, is 12 feet long; many of the other figures are over 6 feet tall.

LA JOLLA

La Jolla Cave: Enter through the Shell Shop, 1325 Coast Boulevard. Open Monday–Friday 10 A.M.–4:30 P.M.; Sunday, 11 A.M.–5 P.M. Admission: $1; children, 50¢. Phone: (619) 454-6080.

For that back-to-the-womb feeling, complete with wet, sloshy noises, enter the stone tunnel. Creep down the 141 steps to the huge sea cave. As you stand safely on a platform at sea level, the water rushes in and out all around you.

LOMA LINDA
(Five miles southeast of San Bernardino)

Embryology Museum: on the Loma Linda Medical School campus, in Shryock Hall (the back of the building faces Stewart Street). Museum is on the main floor, in the Anatomy Department. The receptionist will show you the room. Open June–September, Monday–Thursday, 8 A.M.–noon and 1–5 P.M.; Friday, 8 A.M.–2 P.M. During the school year the museum is closed when classes are held there (usually part of Tuesday and Thursday) but otherwise open the same hours as above; call ahead to make sure of times. Admission: free. Phone: (714) 824-4301.

Loma Linda's collection of embryos and fetuses is among the most extensive in the country, if not the world. Actual embryos at every stage of development—from conception on up—are preserved and displayed in jars of formaldehyde and blocks of plastic. If you're easily upset, stay away from the freak baby section, which includes authentic corpses of babies born with no brains, Siamese twins, and deformities too shocking to describe here. Then again, if you're easily upset, why are you visiting this museum at all?

LONE PINE

Alabama Hills: From downtown Lone Pine, go west on Whitney Portal Road; after about one mile you'll see the beginnings of the hills on both sides of the road. After three miles you'll come to Movie Flat Road, which branches north into part of the hills. You can also continue past Movie Flat Road for one-half mile, turn south on Meadows Road for two miles, and turn east on Tuttle Creek Road back to Lone Pine. This route is known as Picture Rocks Circle. Visible anytime. Admission: free. For more information, call (619) 876-4444.

Hannibal the Cannibal lives in the Alabama Hills. So does the Crooked Lady, Fishman, and Big Bertha. They're not very talkative, but that's understandable considering they're rocks. The bizarre geological formations west of Lone Pine have attracted an endless stream of movie directors making westerns; you've probably seen many of these stones on late-night TV, just over Zorro's shoulder. Other inspired names for some of these crazily shaped monoliths include The Spooks, Peter's Pumpkin, Rhino Feet, and our favorite: Hands from Hades.

NATIONAL CITY
(Just south of San Diego)

Museum of American Treasures: 1315 East 4th Street, near L Avenue, northern side of town. Hours and admission undetermined at press time. For current information, call Shirley Lindemann at (619) 474-6886 or (619) 477-7489.

All glass made before 1914 contained manganese; when left out in the sun, it turned purple. During WWI, manganese was needed for munitions, so the glassmakers had to do without it. Even after the war, manganese was never used in glassmaking again. This museum (which used to go by the more provocative title Halls of Desert Glass) is mostly devoted to one man's collection of over 5,000 pieces of pre-WWI purple glass (including candlesticks, crucifixes, bowls and vases). Over the years more curios were added—an extensive doorstop collection and carved tusks—until the old name no longer applied. The new curator was refurbishing the museum when we visited.

OCEANSIDE

St. Malo: at the extreme southern tip of Oceanside, at the end of Pacific Street, south of where it intersects with Eaton Street, nestled between St. Malo Beach and Buena Vista Lagoon. Never open. No admission. No phone.

St. Malo is an ultra-exclusive, xenophobic private city-within-a-city, founded in the '20s as an enclave for Orange County millionaires and socialites. St. Malo's strict architectural code dictates that all buildings be half-timbered, English Tudor-style mansions. The effect is a startling glimpse into a 16th-century Sussex village, marred only by the BMWs and Bentleys. Your chances of getting in through St. Malo's only entrance gate are rather slim, as a guard usually checks strangers. Your best bet is to walk along Oceanside Beach as far as you can go, and then keep going father onto St. Malo Beach, from which you can see part of the town.

PALM SPRINGS

Naturist B & B: Le Petit Chateau, 1491 Via Soledad, between Palmera and Sonora, south side of town. Reservations required. Room rates: $80–$100. Phone: (619) 325-2686.

The owners of this place are fond of saying that they run their Chateau after the "French Mediterranean tradition." We know what goes on in the Mediterranean, don't we? Everybody's naked. All the time. No; they're not, but here at Le Petit Chateau people are naked. This is the nation's only clothing-optional inn, where guests can lounge around the pool, soak in the hot tub—even belly up to the breakfast table—in the glorious altogether.

RANCHO MIRAGE
(Ten miles southeast of Palm Springs)

Streets of the Stars: in and around Blue Skies Village Mobile Home Park. Just north of Country Club Drive on the east side of Highway 111, west of Morningside Country Club. Always visible. Admission: free. For more information, call Blue Skies Village at (619) 328-2600.

Rancho Mirage does Hollywood one better: Instead of setting stars' names into the sidewalks, they name whole streets after them. A winding route through this small section of town takes you down Bing Crosby Drive, Danny Kaye Road, Greer Garson Road, Claudette Colbert Road, Barbara Stanwyck Road, Jack Benny Road, and Burns and Allen Road (he's the right side of the street; she's the left). Elsewhere in town are Frank

Sinatra Drive, Gerald Ford Drive, and Bob Hope Drive. What—no Fatty Arbuckle Boulevard?

RIALTO

Wigwam Village Motel: 2728 West Foothill Boulevard, at Le Pepper Avenue. Price range: around $35 per night. Phone: (714) 875-0241.

Let's get this straight: Sioux Indians lived in tipis, and Chippewas lived in wigwams. Or was it Arapahos that lived in wigwams, and Cherokees in tipis? Oh, forget it. Who can tell the difference between a wigwam and a tipi, anyway? Certainly not the happy-go-lucky tourists who stay in the 19 cement wigwams here at the Wigwam Village Motel. Don't expect a primitive plains lifestyle: These wigwams, built in 1955, are ultra deluxe (as wigwams go), equipped with all mod cons and queen-sized beds. And make sure that's *tobacco* in your peace pipe.

RIVERSIDE

Castle Amusement Park Miniature Golf: 3500 Polk Street, at Magnolia, just north of Highway 91, southwest end of town. Open Sunday–Thursday, 10 A.M.–10 P.M.; Friday–Saturday, 10 A.M.–midnight. Admission: $4; children and seniors, $3. Phone: (714) 785-4140.

California's lost Spanish mission is right here in Riverside—right near the haunted house, the frontier fort, and the Bavarian castle. Unaccountably, someone had the audacity to build a miniature golf course around the mission. Have they no shame?

Life-Size Model Dinosaurs: Jurupa Mountains Cultural Center, 7621 Granite Hill Drive, just off Highway 60, north of downtown. (Granite Hill Drive is a frontage road for Highway 60. Cultural Center is midway between the Valley Way and Pyrite exits.) Dinosaur tours Saturday, 9 A.M. Admission: $2.25. Phone: (714) 685-5818.

Dinosaurs are sproutin' on the hill, just as regular as Grandma's chrysanthemums. Every year for the past seven years, one visionary man and armies of schoolchildren have spent their summers building dinosaurs here. Winterized telephone poles form the monsters' legs. You'll spot all your favorites: a Stegosaurus, Tyrannosaurus Rex, and more.

SAN DIEGO

Cowboy Museum: 2543 Congress Street, in Old Town. Open daily, 10 A.M.–6:30 P.M. Admission: free. Phone: (619) 295-2614.

A cowboy museum, you say? Then what's that jazz band made of limpet shells doing here? And that plastic moose? Pay them no mind: Turn your attention to the crudely impressionistic mini-dioramas of cowboy scenes, sporting such titles as "Vaquero—from whom the cowboy learned his skills," all crammed into one tiny room next to the gift shop. Yippie ti yi yo.

Hall of Success: 221 Westgate Plaza Mall, which is a passageway running parallel to and half a block north of Broadway between 2nd and 3rd Avenues, downtown San Diego, just north of Horton Plaza Centre; at ground level, next to California Federal Savings. Always visible through the window. Admission: free. Phone: (619) 238-1818.

Portraits of the most successful men in American history are enshrined here...great personages such as George Gildred, president of Gildred Development, and Jerry Craig, head honcho of Jerry Craig International. Never heard of them? Don't worry, neither has anyone else. Hall of Success is actually an ingenious scam by a clever—if not very talented—portrait artist. It's simple: He rents a storefront, dubs it "Hall of Success," advertises it as a portrait museum of famous and successful Americans, and then he contacts egotistical small-time businessmen. "You have the rare honor of being chosen..." and you can guess the rest. For a hefty sum he'll whip out an uninspired portrait and hang it on the wall next to all the other chumps. "Hall of Suckers," perhaps?

Places of Learning: inside Sea World, which is on the southern edge of Mission Bay Park on Sea World Drive, just north of Highway 8 and west of Highway 5. Open daily, 9 A.M.–dusk. Admission to all of Sea World: $19.95; children 3–11, $14.95; children under 3, free. Phone (619) 226-3845.

Forget about killer whales and trained seals—who needs 'em? On Sea World's eastern edge (to the right as you enter the main gate) is the park's most interesting corner, Places of Learning. Ostensibly for kids (as is the rest of Sea World, when you get right down to it), POL's main attraction is a vast, one-acre map of the United States. The Gulf of Mexico and the Great Lakes are actual pools of cool blue water. Off the coast of Florida is a 25-square-foot chessboard with gorgeous four-foot-high pieces, which, frustratingly, can't be moved. Just to the left of the Parents' Store is an English-style hedge maze guarded by six-foot replicas of classic children's books. Hell, you've already shelled out the 20 bucks—you might as well expand your mind.

U.S. Open Sand Sculpture Contest: a Sunday in July, depending on the tides. Building starts at 8:30 A.M.; judging is at 1:30 P.M. On Imperial Beach, south of San Diego in the city of Imperial Beach, near the pier. For current date and more information, call (619) 429-4757 or (619) 424-3151.

Over 150,000 spectators jostle for space to watch 450 competitors on ten-person teams build the most elaborate sand sculptures ever to brave the incoming tide. Among the six categories are Sea Creatures and Best Replica of Anything (for which contestants must show a photo of what they are copying). If you only plan to see one sand sculpture contest, why not see the best?

SKYFOREST
(One mile south of Lake Arrowhead)

Santa's Village: three-quarters of a mile east of town, on the north side of Highway 18. Open mid-June–mid-September, daily, 10 A.M.–5 P.M.; November 11–January 1, daily, 10 A.M.–5 P.M.; second half of September and first half of June, Saturday and Sunday only, 10 A.M.–5 P.M.. Closed rest of year. Admission: $7.50; children under two, free. Phone (714) 337-2481 or (714) 336-3661.

When we were kids, our parents refused to take us to Santa's Village. They didn't believe in Santa, they said. Don't make the same mistake. Climb into a giant ornament and spin around and around a 15-foot Christmas tree, as giant toadstools and candy canes beckon below and Mrs. Claus presides over her Alpine kitchen. A whole theme park dedicated to Santa—you'll never again need to make one of those troublesome journeys to the North Pole! When it's August and you just gotta have a sleigh ride, this is the place to go.

TWENTYNINE PALMS
(50 miles northeast of Palm Springs)

Outhouse Race: first Sunday in October, 2 P.M. On Gorgonio Drive (two blocks north of Highway 62), between Adobe Road and Mesquite Avenue, downtown. For more information, call (619) 367-3445.

Out here in California, we'll race anything. Even outhouses. Each entry requires four pushers and one sitter, and must complete a round-trip circuit up and down the street. The winners of the preliminary heats go on to compete in the championship finals: Finalists are awarded toilet-seat trophies. Smart racers have practice "runs."

VICTORVILLE

Hula-Ville: on Amargosa Road, southwest of Victorville. Exit Highway 15 north at Bear Valley Road and

turn left immediately on Amargosa Road (which is the frontage road to the highway), and go southwest for about 1½ miles. You can also exit at Main Street and turn northeast. Hula-Ville is visible from the road and from the highway. Open daily, daylight hours. Admission: free.

Miles Mahan, desert poet and eccentric landscape architect, lives in a roofless home made of Joshua trees, bottles, and chicken wire. Once a welcomed, wacky vision along Route 66, "Mahan's Half-Acre" of painted signs and junk art was bypassed by the streamlined Highway 15. The visitors are fewer now, yet Mahan still loves to entertain weary travelers with inspired verse and the occasional tap dance. Hula-Ville's mascot is a 12-foot-high hula girl, once a billboard for a now-defunct restaurant. Mahan sticks bottles and cans on every plant and fence post in sight and has fashioned an entire mini-golf driving range among the cacti. His leading passion, though, is painting corny jokes and rhymes on wooden boards. Hundreds of these decorate the property.

Roy Rogers–Dale Evans Museum: 15650 Seneca Road, northeast of downtown. From Highway 15, take the Palmdale Road exit north. Open daily, 9 A.M.–5 P.M. (ticket booth closes at 4:30). Admission: $3; seniors and children 13–16, $2; children 6–12, $1. Phone: (619) 243-4547.

This blend of the absurdly private and the hogwashy Hollywood will leave you puzzled, desperate to figure out which of these artifacts really had meaning for Roy and Dale—for surely some of them did—and which are the counterfeits. It's a bizarre puzzle, and the pieces have something to do with the American West, something to do with the American family, something to do with publicity: $1,000 saddles, pictures of now-dead children, bronzed boots, plaster madonnas, rings made out of $2 bills. What do you make of it? There's a replica of the Rogers' family kitchen. The plates are decorated with broncos and cattle brands. You want to believe the family really ate off these, but.... And there are taxidermed game animals, Roy's mother's doll collection, trash cans shaped like boots, Roy Rogers lunch boxes. Somehow it's very disturbing.

YUCCA VALLEY
(25 miles north of Palm Springs)

Antone Martin Memorial Park: northern end of Mohawk Trail (at Sunnyslope), on the hill above town, just north of Highway 62. Visible anytime. Admission: free. Phone: (619) 365-2376.

Others beat their brows and moan, "Why did Judas betray Jesus?" We beat our brows and moan, "Why'd they change the name of this attraction from Desert Christ Park to Antone Martin Memorial Park?" We all know which name is better. What were they afraid of? Cement, steel, and plaster statues loom on the desert hillside, depicting the Sermon on the Mount, Christ in the House of Lazarus, and other scenes. The 2½-story "Last Supper" bas-relief has a square cut out around Jesus's head, so that the sun- and moonlight can pour through and create a halo effect.

LOS ANGELES AND ORANGE COUNTY

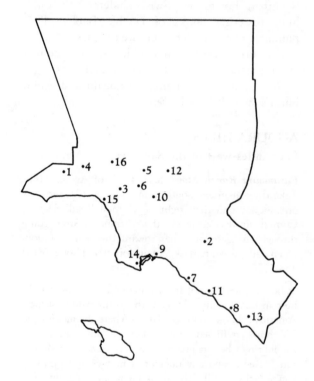

Legend:
1. Agoura Hills
2. Anaheim
3. Beverly Hills
4. Calabasas
5. Glendale
6. Hollywood
7. Huntington Beach
8. Laguna Beach
9. Long Beach
10. Los Angeles
11. Newport Beach
12. Pasadena
13. San Juan Capistrano
14. San Pedro
15. Santa Monica
16. Van Nuys

L.A. is what you dream when you have a fever. The hard heat nagging you summer and winter, squeezing your head into all sorts of odd shapes. The yellow haze around everything. The endless road and the endless squinting into street signs, the endless squealing of car brakes. The squadrons of palm trees forever marching at the edge of your field of vision.

And things here look like other things, no matter how hard you peer at them through the haze. Suburban homes are Swiss chalets, Polynesian huts, towering hunks of Dubble Bubble. Restaurants are castles. Theaters are temples.

Still other things here couldn't sensibly be real at all. Elephantine donuts. UFO worshippers.

You blink your stinging eyes again and again, but it's *there*. It's really *there*.

AGOURA HILLS
(Ten miles west of the San Fernando Valley)

Paramount Ranch Movie Set: south of Agoura Hills. Take the Kanan exit south from Highway 101; turn left on Sideway and then right on Cornell Road. Stay on Cornell until you reach the entrance. After going through the gate, turn left toward the ranger station. Open daily, dawn to dusk. Admission: free. Phone: (818) 888-3770.

The wild west is not in Arizona or Nevada, but right here in L.A. County. At least, this is the wild west most Americans know and love. This is where the movies and TV shows are filmed. The sets here at Paramount Ranch should ring a bell in anyone who's ever seen "Bat Masterson," "Reds," and any number of movies and shows. If you're lucky, you'll arrive on a day when some filming is going on. The sets are still very much in use.

Renaissance Pleasure Faire: six weekends in late April and May; usually the last weekend or two in April and all the weekends in May. Paramount Ranch, south of Agoura Hills. Take the Kanan exit south from Highway 101; turn left on Sideway and then right on Cornell Road. Stay on Cornell until you reach the entrance of Paramount Ranch. Signs and parking attendants guide you the rest of the way. Admission: $14.50; seniors, $11.50; children, $7.50. Phone: (213) 202-8854.

The faire, in theory, is a historically accurate re-creation of a 16th-century English market village. Thousands of authentically costumed actors, merchants, and craftspeople play host to not-so-authentically costumed tourists amid rolling hills, oaks, and booths and stages built to 16th-century specifications. The event's main shortcoming is that the admirable efforts of the employees to create a historically accurate environment are squelched by the sheer number of shorts-wearing, sunglassed Angelenos blanketing the landscape like locusts. In the "good old days"—say, ten or 20 years ago—many tourists came in costume and became part of the show. We recommend that you dress appropriately. It's more fun that way.

ALTADENA

Banana Museum: open by appointment only. Admission: free. To make an appointment and get directions, call (818) 798-2272.

A whole bunch of banana trinketry fills this, the official museum of the International Banana Club. It's the consuming hobby of Ken Bannister, who calls himself Bananister and who thinks bananas look like smiles. Club members from all over the world have donated the artifacts: giant rubber bananas; banana liqueurs; banana greeting cards; banana cereals, baby foods, and jellos; toy monkeys holding bananas; a banana Christmas tree; banana shirts....At last count, the museum housed over 10,000 items. Keep your eyes peeled.

ANAHEIM

Theme Motels: The birth of Disneyland gave an entrepreneur named Stovall the idea to open a chain of theme motels nearby. Stovall is long gone, but most of his motels remain. Here are three of the best.

Stovall's Inn/Wonderland of Topiary Trees: 1110 West Katella Avenue. Visible anytime. Phone: (714) 778-1880.
They don't make motels like they used to. This motel's theme is topiary, the nearly lost art of molding living bushes to look like animals, ice-cream cones...anything but bushes. Stovall's topiary tends toward the cartoony-animal 1950s style, in deference to a certain amusement park across the street. Ten-foot topiary elephants march along on their hind legs; other pachyderms throw back their heads and laugh uproariously. There's also a gaggle of Santa's reindeer (impressive antlers), llamas, giraffes,

"wild stallions," a moose, a rocking horse, and a humanoid rabbit.

Fabulous Space Age Lodge: 1176 West Katella Avenue. Visible anytime. Phone: (714) 776-0141.

This was Stovall's space-age theme motel. Unfortunately, Best Western, the motel's new owner, toned down the spaciness. God knows why. Still here are geometric metal "satellites" on the roof, 1950s-style "atoms" perched atop poles, a geodesic-dome pool shack, and, of course, an astronaut on the sign. The pool is shaped sort of like a space re-entry capsule. A row of merry topiary hippos romps at poolside. Other vegetable animals dot the grounds, though most are not in as good condition as the ones at Stovall's Inn.

Apollo Inn: 1741 South West Street. Visible anytime. Phone: (714) 772-9750.

Next door to the Disneyland Motel is the somewhat themeless Apollo Inn. But still, it has its own bushy menagerie of topiary critters, all in pretty clip-top condition. The Monorail glides overhead.

* * * *

White House Replica and Hobby City Doll and Toy Museum: 1238 South Beach Boulevard, between Ball Road and Cerritos Avenue. Open daily, 10 A.M.–6 P.M. Admission: $1; children under 12 and seniors, 50¢. Phone: (714) 527-2323.

This exact half-sized replica of the White House was built, say its owners, so that visitors "could walk through the same doors that the world's most important people have walked through." Inside are over 3,000 dolls of all kinds, including a 4,000-year-old specimen that was found in an Egyptian pyramid. Remember: This is only a replica. Those dolls are not the president.

ARCADIA

L.A. State and County Arboretum: 301 North Baldwin Avenue, just north of Huntington Drive and just south of Highway 210 (the Foothill Freeway), adjacent to Santa Anita Racetrack. Open daily, 9 A.M.–4:30 P.M. Admission: $3; students and seniors, $1.50; children 5–12, 75¢; children under 5, free. Phone (818) 446-8257.

Remember those good feelings you had while watching *Attack of the Giant Leeches?* The tingles you got while watching *Cannibal Attack* and *Waikiki Wedding?* Relive those moments. Visit the place where these and 50 years' worth of other greats were filmed. The 127-acre arboretum has an African section, South American section, Mediterranean section, North American/Asiatic section, and Australian section. (The Australian section is where the African scenes in "Roots" were filmed. There's reality for you.) Also here are a Prehistoric Garden (sorry, no dinosaurs: only plants), Aquatic Garden, Herb Garden, and more.

BEVERLY HILLS

The Beverly Hills Annual Waiters' and Waitresses' Race: first Sunday in December, starting about 9 A.M., at Beverly Hills High School, near Olympic Boulevard and Spalding Drive. Finish line is also at Beverly Hills High School. For more information, call (213) 550-4816.

In France, racing waiters and waitresses balance a bottle of beer on a tray as they run. But not in Beverly Hills, oh no. Beverly Hills waiters must balance a bottle of *Perrier*. They have to run a whole five kilometers through the backroads of Beverly Hills, not just up and down the block. Black-and-white waiterly garb is de rigeur, too, not to mention courtesy and correct posture. Give 'em a break. Bring a picnic lunch.

Counter Spy Shop: 9465 Wilshire Boulevard, Room 210, second floor. Open Monday–Friday, 9 A.M.–5 P.M. Phone: (213) 274-6256.

World-famous authors like ourselves are plagued by spies out to steal our literary secrets. They tap our phones, hoping to overhear witticisms tumbling from our lips; they photograph our manuscripts as we stroll blithely to the copy shop; they cook up elaborate schemes to steal our typewriters. That's why we need the Counter Spy Shop. They manufacture and sell "security" devices you thought existed only in the pages of espionage novels. The selection ranges from bulletproof cars with hidden gun ports and antikidnapping alarm transmitters to mini-safes hidden in Pepsi cans. A specialty here is antibugging devices. Our favorites were the see-in-the-dark binoculars and the parabolic microphone that can actually pick up conversations one mile away.

Hollywood On Location: 8644 Wilshire Boulevard, near Carson Road. Open Monday-Friday, 9:30 A.M.–4:30 P.M.

Price: $29 for complete list and maps. Phone: (213) 659-9165.

It's every stargazer's dream come true: a complete list of every single site in L.A. where TV shows and movies are being filmed on any given day. That's what your $29 buys. You also get maps showing exact locations, a list of stars (and nobodies) who will be appearing, and extra tidbits such as the exact time of filming and type of scene (stunt, chase, etc.). They'll even let you take a sneak preview before you pay, to see if any of your favorite stars are on the list. It's a good idea to show up early, or make advance reservations, as they print up only a limited number of lists. On the day we visited, the list featured 30 "shoots", and Chevy Chase, O. J. Simpson, Tony Curtis, Vanna White, and Anne Bancroft were appearing.

The Scriptorium: 427 North Canon Drive, #112 in the Courtyard mini-mall. Hours are variable. Phone: (213) 275-6060 or (213) 278-4200.

This little shop, basking in the mellow glow of old papers, is an autograph gallery. Scribbles of the rich and famous—beauties, bandleaders, and bards—are here, with price tags in the thousands and tens of thousands of dollars. Didn't bring your checkbook? You're still welcome to peruse the John Hancocks of Eleanor Roosevelt, Abbott and Costello, Susan B. Anthony, and hundreds more.

Willat Studios Building: at the corner of Walden Drive and Carmelita Avenue, at the 500 block of Walden. Always visible from the outside.

Also known as "The Witch House," this pointy-roofed anomaly was built in Culver City, moved to Beverly Hills, and is now scheduled for a move back to Culver City. Most famous for its appearance in the movie *The Loved One*, Willat Studios' inspiration comes from the world of scary bedtime stories. Ragged, weathered shingles cover absurdly steep gables; strangely asymmetrical shutters frame the half-wooded windows; an old streetlight stands in the front yard. A mock pier named Witch's Landing stands in an imaginary lake. If the house is missing when you arrive, inquire in Culver City.

BUENA PARK

Medieval Times: 7662 Beach Boulevard, one long block north of Knott's Berry Farm. Open for free, self-guided walking tours Monday–Saturday, 9 A.M.–4 P.M. Dinner/performances held nightly. In summer: two seatings Monday–Saturday, 6 and 8:45 P.M.; three seatings Sunday, 1, 4:45, and 7:30 P.M. In winter, one seating Monday–Thursday, 7:30 P.M.; two seatings Friday and Saturday, 6:15 and 9 P.M.; Sunday, 1, 4:45, and 7:30 P.M. Admission to dinner/shows: $24–$28; children 12 and under, $16–$18. Phone: outside California, (800) 826-5358, or in California, (800) 438-9911.

First of all, there's this castle in Buena Park. Every night, a few thousand diners fill the arenalike seats, cheer their favorite jousters, pay loud homage to an 11th-century Spanish count, and tear roast chickens limb from limb with their bare hands. (Heck, you should see what they do to the chocolate creampuffs.) Fully costumed horsemen, using real swords, maces, and ten-foot lances, have everybody gasping as they joust, ride-at-the-ring, and otherwise revive spine-tingling medieval sports. The shining-bearded MC, the "wenches" and "serfs" who serve the meal, and the skilled jousters never slip out of character, which is refreshing.

CALABASAS

Pet Cemetery: 5068 North Old Scandia Lane. From Highway 101 (Ventura Freeway), take the Calabasas Parkway exit (north) and turn right to Ventura Boulevard. Old Scandia Lane branches north off Ventura. Open Monday–Saturday, 8 A.M.–5 P.M.; Sunday 11 A.M.–3 P.M. Admission: free. Phone: (818) 347-7037.

Who owns and maintains this 10-acre cemetery, with its 40,000 little mounds wherein sleep 50 years' worth of loyal pals? A group called S.O.P.H.I.E.—Save Our Pets' History In Eternity—that's who. Thus you can expect a lion's share of sentimentality here. Many gravestones sport ceramicized photos of the deceased. On (or in or under) the premises are Hopalong Cassidy's horse; the Little Rascals' dog; pets of Gloria Swanson and Rudolf Valentino; and herds, gaggles, and packs of other dead pets.

CLAREMONT

The Fiske Museum of Musical Instruments: Bridges Auditorium, in the Claremont University Center, corner of 4th and College Way. Open Monday, Wednesday, and Friday, 2–4 P.M.; Tuesday and Thursday, 10 A.M.–noon.

Also open by appointment. Admission: free. Phone: (714) 621-8307.

Even if you don't know how to play an over-the-shoulder saxhorn, you can get a good look at one in this museum. Also here are Tibetan temple trumpets, experimental instruments, Asian lutes, and a seven-foot trumpet—the world's largest.

COSTA MESA

Museum of Historical Documents: 3333 Bear Street (at Sunflower), on the third floor, one block west of South Coast Plaza Mall. Open Monday–Friday, 10 A.M.–9 P.M.; Saturday, 10 A.M.–6 P.M.; Sunday, 11 A.M.–6 P.M. Admission: free. Phone: (714) 662-2255.

Psst—wanna buy a letter? It's only $35,000. Signed by Abraham Lincoln. That's just a sample of the merchandise at this museum/shop, whose archives hold all of 72,000 documents and letters signed by famous people. The oldest in the collection is a scribble from Ferdinand and Isabella of Spain. All over the walls you can see framed signatures of entertainers, politicians, artists, and even villains.

GLENDALE

Forest Lawn: 1712 South Glendale Avenue, southern edge of the city. Open daily, 9 A.M.–5 P.M. Admission: free. Phone: (818) 241-4151.

Hey, don't call it a cemetery. Thousands of rotting corpses lie mould'ring in the grave as you wander past enthusiastic replicas of every patriotic and classical structure from here to Vatican City. Don't miss the Wee Kirk O' the Heather; the stained-glass "Last Supper" window (taped narrative repeats on the half-hour); the Freedom Mausoleum (urns 'n' patriotic statues); the replica of Michelangelo's David; and the Court of Freedom, full of re-created scenes from the revolution (ours). An eclectic museum has replicas of the British Crown Jewels, an Easter Island head, and an example of every coin mentioned in the Bible.

HANCOCK PARK

International Festival of Masks: last weekend in October, noon–dusk. Parade of Masks starts at 11:30 A.M.

Sunday and goes down Wilshire between Curson Street and Crescent Heights Boulevard. Rest of festival takes place in Hancock City Park, Wilshire Boulevard between Ogden and Curson Streets. Visitors are encouraged to wear masks. For more information, call (213) 934-8527.

Wanna lose face? Head for the mask festival. A masked parade, mask-making workshops, and continuous masked entertainment (e.g., folk dancing) bring out false faces of every color, shape, and nationality. Lecturers explore the cultural significance of masks, and mask-makers sell their wares.

HOLLYWOOD

Aetherius Society Headquarters: 6202 Afton Place, four blocks from Sunset and Vine. Open normal business hours, plus variable additional hours on weekends and evenings. Admission: free. Phone: (213) 465-9652 or (213) 467-4325.

In May 1954, an Englishman on the verge of an emotional breakdown started hearing voices that said to him, "Prepare yourself! You are to become the Voice of Interplanetary Parliament!" No, he didn't end up in an asylum. He ended up in L.A., as the leader of a highly successful UFO cult. The Aetherius Society's belief system is outlandish and convoluted. "Cosmic Masters"—including Krishna, Buddha, Jesus, and two beings named Aetherius and Mars Sector 6—come from outer space in spaceships to visit our planet periodically, to help humans graduate from "classroom earth." (Jesus comes from Venus. He last showed up in 1958.) Aetherians believe in channeling, reincarnation, UFOs, and yoga. They spend their time charging up prayer batteries and placating the Lords of the Ineffable Flame of Terra. Their headquarters has a display area and bookstore, which you may visit. But keep these caveats in mind: (1) Act honestly interested. (2) Don't giggle. (3) Be prepared. (4) Don't take photographs. May the Cosmic Masters be with you!

Bra Museum: in the Frederick's of Hollywood store, 6608 Hollywood Boulevard, between Highland and Cahuenga. Open Monday–Thursday, 10 A.M.–8 P.M.; Friday, 10 A.M.–9 P.M.; Saturday, 10 A.M.–6 P.M.; Sunday, noon–5 P.M. Admission: free. Phone: (213) 466-8506.

Bras and bosoms get the historical treatment here as bra blueprints, advertisements, and actual specimens dating from 1946 to the present march proudly along. Pointette, Bright Light, and Depth Charge are names of unsubtle 1950s bras. The later-vintage Sexposé model has this advice to recommend it: "Bare your nipples but be smart and put your breasts on a shelf!!" And Hollywood would be one dull burg without the bras of the stars. On view here are Mamie Van Doren's surprisingly archaic one, Isabel Sanford's enormous one, and Madonna's scary one, as well as bras worn by famous men.

Dudley Do-Right's Emporium: 8200 Sunset Boulevard, at Havenhurst, on the border of West Hollywood. Open Tuesday–Thursday, 10 A.M.–5 P.M. Phone: (213) 656-6550.

Saturday morning cartoon scholars agree that the man responsible for the wittiest, most socially aware, and most slyly sophisticated cartoons is Jay Ward. He's responsible for Rocky and Bullwinkle; Natasha and Boris; Superchicken; Dudley Do-Right; and George, George, George of the Jungle. You can get Walt Disney paraphernalia just about anywhere, but this place is one of the few that sells Jay Ward accoutrements: not just T-shirts, either, but also aprons, buttons, rubber stamps, cards, dolls, refrigerator magnets, and the most popular item of all, painted scene cells from the original cartoons. Watch out for that tree!

Forest Lawn Hollywood Hills: 6300 Forest Lawn Drive, just west of Griffith Park and just south of Highway 134 (the Ventura Freeway). Open daily, 9 A.M.–5 P.M. Admission: free. Phone: (818) 984-1711.

Where do you go when you need a quick religio-patriotic fix? A reminder that "God gave us our liberty, and people who forsake God lose their liberty"? To the graveyard, that's where. At Forest Lawn you'll find an Old North Church replica; a 26-minute film called *The Birth of Liberty*; and the nation's largest historical mosaic, made of 10 million bits of Venetian glass. Also here is the Plaza of Mexican Heritage, home to replicas of pre-Columbian statuary, desert plants, and a Mexican history museum. Don't leave the cemetery without learning the mathematical secrets of the Mayas.

Grave Line Tours: departs daily at noon from the corner of Hollywood Boulevard and Orchid Avenue, along the east wall of Mann's Chinese Theater. Admission: $25; advance reservation, $30. Phone: (213) 392-5501.

Cozily ensconced in a silver hearse, you careen past the scenes of Hollywood's greatest demises. The hilarious and well-researched taped narrative provides exuberant blow-by-blow accounts of over 70 fascinating deaths. During the ride a few myths are dispelled (note to Mama Cass fans: It was *not* a ham sandwich) and a few choice bits of nondeath gossip are proffered (note to "I Love Lucy" fans: Vivian Vance's contract stipulated that she remain 20 pounds overweight for the duration of the show). Learn about Paul Lynde's final fling, Sharon Tate's last meal....

Hollywood in Miniature: 6843 Hollywood Boulevard, across the street from Mann's Chinese Theater, inside a gift shop called On Location Hollywood. Open Sunday–Thursday, 8 A.M.–11 P.M.; Friday–Saturday, 8 A.M.–1 A.M. Admission: $2.50; children under 12, free with adult. Phone: (213) 466-7758.

Is this nearly 50-year-old precise 3-D model of Hollywood a labor of love or the product of an incurable obsessive-compulsive? Perhaps a little of both. Originally it thrived as a boardwalk sideshow in Atlantic City, where starry-eyed easterners got a glimpse of the legendary Tinseltown. Now, after a four-decade appointment with a forgotten warehouse, Hollywood in Miniature has been rediscovered and reinstalled in—of all places—Hollywood. God forbid the Russians should get ahold of this. Then they'd know what Hollywood is like, down to the number of fronds on every palm tree. Our national security could be jeopardized. But wait—this is how Hollywood looked in the '40s! Don't you think that's a little out of date? Okay, Vladimir, here's your ticket. Enjoy your visit.

Max Factor Beauty Museum: 1666 North Highland Avenue, one-half block south of the 6700 block of Hollywood Boulevard. Open Monday–Saturday, 10 A.M.–4 P.M. Admission: free. Phone: (213) 463-6668.

Whether you worship Hollywood's version of beauty or think it's an instrument of the devil, you'll find plenty to amuse you here. Don't miss the plastic lip machine, designed to check the adhesion powers of various lipsticks. Or the Beauty Calibrator, a 1932 face-measuring device that looks like an Iron Maiden. Also here are the world's first human-hair wig and hairpieces worn by George Burns, Jimmy Stewart, Frank Sinatra, and Lucille Ball. Photos illustrate the grotesque art of wigmaking. Another snapshot shows Natalie Wood without makeup, looking like a nice normal person, someone you might see on the bus.

Motion Picture Coordination Office: 6922 Hollywood Boulevard, near Sycamore Avenue, in the Hollywood Center Building, sixth floor, room 600. (Turn left after exiting elevator.) Open Monday–Friday, 10:30 A.M.–5 P.M. (sometimes 11:30 A.M.–5 P.M. on busy days). Price: free, if you copy down the information yourself; $1 plus 10¢ per page if you want a photocopy. Phone: (213) 485-5324.

At Hollywood on Location (See Beverly Hills) it costs you $29 to find out where movies and TV shows are being filmed on any given day; here you can get the same information for free. What's the difference (besides the money)? Hollywood on Location gives maps and more details; the Motion Picture Coordination Office supplies a rudimentary list with little more information than the name of what's being filmed and an address. Still, this free service actually lists more "shoots" and includes commercials, stills, and videos. You're definitely taking your chances with flicks like *I'mo Git You Sucka-Feat* and *Far Out, Man!* but at this price who's complaining?

Sarno's Caffé Dell' Opera: 1714 North Vermont, at Prospect. Open Sunday–Thursday, 5 P.M.–11 P.M.; Friday–Saturday, 5 P.M.–midnight. Singing usually starts around 9 P.M. Price: moderate. Phone: (213) 662-3403.

Hey, all you would-be Carusos, come out of the shower. Anyone—well, let's be honest: anyone with a little talent—can get up from his plate of tortellini to belt out a few *O Sole Mios* and *Figaros*, to the wild applause of his fellow diners. Founded by Alberto Sarno, an Italian singer and cook, Sarno's has become a hangout for L.A.-area opera buffs and struggling tenors.

Siamese Castle: 4857 Melrose Avenue, 1½ blocks east of Western Avenue. Outside is visible anytime; restaurant is open Sunday–Thursday, 11:30 A.M.–11 P.M.; Friday, 11:30 A.M.–midnight; Saturday, 4 P.M.–midnight. Phone: (213) 460-6738.

"What will you eat, milady Guinevere?" "Coconut-chicken rad-na and a mug o' Thai iced tea." On the outside, it's a stately English castle. On the inside, it's a Thai restaurant. Most likely, a long-gone architect designed the castle for a now-long-gone, if more relevant, business. Or maybe Anna *did* marry the King of Siam after all.

A Star Is Worn: 7303 Melrose Avenue (at Poinsettia Place), just west of La Brea Avenue. Open Monday–Saturday, 11 A.M.–7 P.M.; Sunday, noon–5 P.M. Phone: (213) 939-4922.

When is a sweatsuit more than just a sweatsuit? When it's Victoria Principal's nearly-new sweatsuit, on sale here for $55. All the clothes, shoes, purses, and trinkets in this second-hand boutique come from the closets of celebrities, both male and female. We saw Suzanne Pleshette's baseball jacket, Joni Mitchell's suede purse (a bit 1970s for our taste), Melissa Gilbert's white gown...and lots of satin, lots of sequins, lots of fame. Each garment comes with a tag identifying its famous former owner.

HUNTINGTON BEACH

International Surfing Museum: at press time, the museum was due to move to new quarters in downtown Huntington Beach, near the pier. Admission: free. For new address and hours, call (714) 536-0155.

Even hodads are welcome to trip out on the surfboards, surf movie posters, surf records, swim trunks, and other memorabilia on display here. Where else but Huntington, one of southern California's totally awesomest beaches, could you see the first guitar ever owned by Dick Dale, and heirloom receipts from surfboard shops of the 1960s? It's rad.

INGLEWOOD

Big Donut: Randy's Donuts, 805 West Manchester Boulevard, at the corner of La Cienega Boulevard. Open daily, 24 hours.

L.A., at one point in its glorious history, was awash in monstrous donuts. Now the few that remain are too stale to eat. Randy's rooftop morsel isn't the biggest in the world; but considering its prime location a few yards from the endless traffic of the San Diego Freeway, it's probably the best known.

LAGUNA BEACH

Pageant of the Masters: early July–late August, nightly at 8:30 P.M., in conjunction with the Festival of the Arts. Irvine Bowl Park, 650 Laguna Canyon Road (shuttle buses run to and from downtown Laguna Beach until midnight). Tickets by reservation only. Price: $9–$35. Phone: (714) 494-1145.

Help! It's a 40-foot Norman Rockwell painting, attacking the Irvine Bowl! Everybody, run! The Pageant of the Masters is a two-hour series of *tableaux vivants*—"living pictures"—in which live human beings "act out" great works of art. Costumes, makeup, painted backgrounds, and fancy lighting tricks, as well as the actors' incredible ability to hold perfectly still for minutes at a time (you actually can't see them breathing), make this an effective, surreal show. You have to keep reminding yourself the figures are human as they act out not just paintings but tapestries, sculptures—even earthenware tiles.

LA PUENTE

Big Donuts: The Donut Hole, 15300 East Amar Road (at Hacienda Boulevard). Open daily, 24 hours. Phone: (818) 968-2912.

Not one but two huge donuts greet you at this 1950s-era drive-thru. Sure, the donuts are oddly smooth and look more like inner tubes. Sure, they're half sunk in the ground. But that's *part of the plan*. See, these are *drive-thru donuts*. You get to drive right through the holes. Oooh.

LONG BEACH

Sand Castle Contest: usually the first or second Sunday in August, as part of Sea Festival. At the foot of Junipero Avenue, on the beach in front of Bixby Park. Contest starts at 9 A.M.; judging at 1:30 P.M. For more information and exact date, call (213) 429-6310.

This well-attended affair grants contestants a long time to pile up their masterpieces, so highly imaginative creations are the order of the day.

LOS ANGELES

Big Donut: on top of Kindle's Donuts, 10003 South Normandie Avenue, at Century Boulevard. Open daily, 24 hours. Phone: (213) 756-8548.

Come and pay homage to the great donut god. Cinnamon-brown and studded with authentic little bumps, this giant donut looms grandly above an uncaring populace.

Clifton's Brookdale Cafeteria: 648 South Broadway, at 7th. Open daily, 6 A.M.–8 P.M. Phone: (213) 627-1673.

"Pay what you wish...dine free unless delighted" reads Clifton's credo—and it's no empty promise, either. You really *can* pay whatever you want for the food, though there are "suggested prices"—generally so low you'd be embarrassed to pay less anyway. This is one of the last remaining 1930s-style cafeterias in California. The outside is gritty; but inside, amazingly, are babbling brooks, waterfalls, bridges, wishing wells, murals, and mosaics of wilderness scenes. There's even a chapel on the upper level. The whole place is done up in a rustic redwood-log theme. And don't forget to read the nutty "Food for Thot" pamphlets, available for free in the cafeteria.

Day of the Dead Celebration: November 2, Olvera Street, downtown. Activities begin around 1 P.M. and last till evening. Altar is set up in front of the historic Avila Adobe. For more information, call (213) 628-7833.

Day of the Dead (*Día de los Muertes*) is a centuries-old Mexican holiday in which the beloved dead are honored

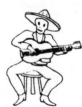

and remembered with macabre joy: Mariachi bands wear skeleton costumes; families picnic at their loved ones' graves: children munch candy skulls with their own names written on top. Olvera Street celebrates with costumes, street theater, skeleton decor, and *muchísimas* candy skulls. At the outdoor altar, people set up photos of dead relatives along with the dead ones' favorite foods and flowers.

Flying Saucer House: 7776 Torreyson Drive. To get there, get onto Mulholland Drive from Hollywood or Studio City. Drive to Torreyson Place, go half a block, and turn right on Torreyson Drive. Go equipped with a map—just in case. Visible anytime, but remember that this is private property.

The most extraordinary private residence in Los Angeles is about as inaccessible as a house can get. The best views of it are from Mulholland Drive or down at the bottom of its long off-limits private driveway on Torreyson Drive. (The problem with Mulholland is that there's nowhere to park; you might try parking at the nearby Universal Studios Overlook and walking from there.) The house looks like an octagonal UFO that has just landed in the Santa Monica Mountains. It's supported by eight steel poles that converge to a point, and it seems to be actively engaged in a game of chicken with the laws of gravity.

Holyland Exhibition: 2215 Lake View Avenue at the corner of Allesandro Way in a square white building, in the Silverlake district. Open daily, but by appointment only; call and they will tell you when tours are being given, and you can choose which tour you want. Admission: $2.50; children under 16, $2 (includes refreshments). Phone: (213) 664-3162.

Pretend that Indiana Jones was a devout Christian. Pretend he saved for his private collection all the rare discoveries he made while searching for the Ark. Pretend he invented wacky religious gimmicks like the Eyeographic Bible Study System, and that a cult grew up around him after his death. Change the name Indiana Jones to Antonio Futterer, and what you've got is the Holyland Bible Knowledge Society, caretakers of the Holyland Exhibition. What you'll see here is a stunning collection of Near Eastern art and artifacts. The tour guide, dressed as a Bedouin, acts nonchalant as she shows off a collection that she may or may not know is worth at least several million dollars. At the end you get to sample Holyland refreshments. Take this chance to inspect the case containing the possibly miraculous cross-shaped tree. A plaque reads, "A perfect *cross* found growing in our front garden Easter 1936. This appeared in Ripley's Believe it or Not   PROVIDENTIAL!"

Kong Chow Temple: 930 North Broadway, in Chinatown. Open daily, 11 A.M.–4 P.M. Admission: free. Phone: (213) 626-1955.

The scene here is straight out of a Dashiell Hammett story, not a Raymond Chandler potboiler. What's a San

Francisco-style Chinese temple doing in L.A.? Well, just because it's in L.A. doesn't mean this Chinatown must be all ranch-style adobes and Mayan-influenced apartment buildings. A Chinatown looks like a Chinatown whether it's in California, Paris, or Australia. So follow the incense up the stairs to the small temple filled with red and gold banners and tapestries, fruit and incense offerings, and plenty of devout Buddhists and Taoists. Be respectful—you know, "Come on, Jake, it's Chinatown."

Mayan Theater: 1040 South Hill Street, near 11th Street. Open whenever movies are being shown, which is pretty much all the time. Outside is visible anytime. Phone: (213) 749-6294.

Yet another eccentric Los Angeles landmark on the skids. Built in 1927, this is probably the largest, most detailed, and most elaborate Mayan-style building erected since the days of the Conquistadores. It once rivaled Grauman's Chinese Theater as L.A.'s most grandly exotic, ethnic-themed theater. But now it shows only Mexican porno films. The outside has four full stories of multicolored Mayan motifs, animal and snake heads and bold geometrics. The only anthropogical boo-boos we found were Mayan chiefs wearing Sioux headdresses. Those of you with nerves of steel and a working knowledge of Spanish obscenities can pay your money and inspect the heavily decorated interior.

Museum of Neon Art: 704 Traction Avenue, downtown. Traction is just off Alameda Street, between 1st and 3rd Streets. Open Tuesday–Saturday, 11 A.M.–5 P.M. Admission: $2.50; students, $1; children under 16, free.

We thought this was going to be a cute, historical collection of vintage neon signs: rocking martini glasses, dancing spurs, all blinking on and off...yay! But MONA, as acronym-lovin' Angelenos call this place, turned out to be changing exhibits of art made with neon. Real art. The kind we can't understand. Boo.

The Next Stage: Tour dates, times, and prices vary. For more information, call (213) 939-2688.

This offbeat tour company offers the Insomniac Tour, which departs 3 A.M. of a Saturday and rambles through the sleeping city till 9 A.M., stopping in the predawn at the L.A. Produce Market, a bagel factory, and more. The company also features a women's history tour of L.A., exploring the haunts of Aimee Semple McPherson and other *femmes fameux*.

Pet Blessing: the Saturday before Easter. Plaza Church, North Main Street, two blocks from Olvera Street, downtown. For exact time and other information, call (213) 687-4344.

Hundreds of pet owners show up, animals in tow, to have the padre bless the critters and thank them for serving humankind. Horses, birds, cats, dogs—even pigs and cows—join in the sanctified fun. Humans are required to keep animals on a leash to cut down on fighting.

The Teapot: 607 West Manchester, near Hoover Street. Always visible from outside. Phone: (213) 973-4848.

Once a quaint teahouse, this teapot-shaped building currently houses Autos Unlimited, a ramshackle auto parts shop. Now in a rundown neighborhood and missing its spout and handle, The Teapot symbolizes the sad fate of L.A.'s formerly proud heritage of eccentric architecture. The few buildings that don't fall prey to mall-happy developers succumb to neglect or misuse as the neighborhoods around them slowly go down the drain.

MANHATTAN BEACH

Sand Castle Contest: last Sunday in July, after the completion of the surfing competition. On Manhattan Beach near the pier. For more information, call (213) 545-4502.

This contest has a definite surf-scene bent, since it's part of Manhattan Beach's Surf Festival.

MARINA DEL REY

Turtle Races: Thursday nights, 9:30 P.M.–midnight, at Brennan's, 4089 Lincoln Boulevard (just south of Washington Boulevard). Nine races per night. Phone: (213) 821-6622.

Living so close to so many yachts with names like *Half-Fast* and E-Z Cum makes patrons of this tavern desperate to amuse themselves in strange ways. Rent a turtle here or bring your own. Place it in the 20-foot circular racetrack...and stand back and watch the action!

MONROVIA

Aztec Hotel: 311 West Foothill Boulevard, at Magnolia. Visible anytime. Phone: (818) 762-1234.

Los Angeles has had its share of architectural crazes, but few were as exotic as the Mayan and Aztec revivals in the 1920s. This residential hotel, designed by Robert Stacy-Judd, was, as far as anybody can tell, the first building in the United States based on Central American designs. The overall concept is more Mayan than Aztec; but, explains the current owner, "Aztec Hotel was a more memorable name." Abstract, raised designs march across the outside walls, making the hotel look for all the world like the tomb of ancient Mexican royalty. Pillars in the lobby are intricately carved, as are the light fixtures. Stained-glass windows and abstract Mayan paintings add to the overwhelming effect.

House in a Reservoir: near Grand and Hillcrest at the northern edge of Monrovia. Never open. No admission. No phone.

We can't reveal the complete address, as the owner insisted we keep the directions vague to weed out the half-hearted rubberneckers. If you're truly interested in seeing a house built inside a waterless reservoir, a uniquely strange design in a city full of strange designs, you're going to have to do a little detective work of your own, prowling around trying to find it. The roof is just a few feet above ground level. The living area sits in what can best be described as a huge cereal bowl set into the ground. The inside is unusual too, but we won't tantalize you with a description. Let's just say you're on your own with this one: It's there, it's weird, but the rest is classified.

NEWPORT BEACH

Character Boat Parade: usually the first Sunday in August. Newport Harbor area, noon–4 P.M. Judging is usually at 4 P.M. For more information, call (714) 644-8211.

Boat owners decorate their crafts with wild and woolly interpretations of a given theme—which might be Space Travel or Fame or Food. Spectators line the shore to watch the more than 100 costumed boats as they cruise the harbor. Prizes for best decor are awarded at the end of the day.

Magic Island: 3505 Via Oporto, on Lido Isle, just south of where Newport Boulevard intersects Pacific Coast Highway. Open for dinner/shows Wednesday–Saturday, 6 P.M.–midnight (varies); brunch/shows Sunday, 9:30 A.M.–2:15 P.M. Show only (no food): Sunday, 2:30 P.M. Admission: dinner/brunch shows, $18–$25; Sunday show only, $10; children, $5. Visitors must be 21 or over (except on Sunday) and must adhere to a dress code. Phone: (714) 675-0900.

Magicians of all kinds leap about, doing tricks while you dine: pulling things out of hats, sawing things in half, making things disappear. Now, Mr. Magician, about our bill....

Newport Harbor Sand Castle Contest: third Sunday in October, at Corona Del Mar State Beach. Contest starts at 10 A.M.; judging is around noon. For more information, call (714) 644-8211.

This sand castle contest is more elaborate than most, occasionally featuring creations made with structural supports.

NORTH HOLLYWOOD

House of Canes and Walking Sticks: 5628 Vineland Avenue, just off Burbank Boulevard. Open Tuesday–Saturday, 10 A.M.–6 P.M. Admission: free. Phone: (818) 769-4007, or outside California, (800) 451-0745.

Okay, so you don't have a limp. But this factory and shop, one of a very few of its kind, is like a museum. Burt Reynolds, Katherine Hepburn, and Bing Crosby have all been customers here, and we wonder which were their choices: the rhinestone-studded walking stick, the one that conceals five brandy flasks, the one with a delicate watch and pillbox set into its head, or the one that conceals a deadly sword. Most interesting of all is a discontinued model: a walking stick made from the stretched-out penis of a bull.

ORANGE

The Orange County Dental Society Museum: 295 South Flower Street, next to the intersection of Highway 5 and Highway 22. Museum is never officially open, but if you walk into the office anytime Monday–Friday, 9

A.M.–5 P.M., they'll let you see the museum. Admission: free. Phone: (714) 542-8808.

You think a trip to the dentist is bad *now*, huh? Just imagine what it was like in days of yore, back before they knew X-rays were bad for you, back in the days of wooden teeth and pliers, back *before anesthesia*. One thing they did have back then was a nice sense of design, so in addition to old dental tools and dentures and drills, you'll see elegant old dentists' chairs and cabinets, classy—though probably deadly—old X-ray machines, and other torture implements.

PACIFIC PALISADES

Self-Realization Fellowship Lake Shrine: 17190 Sunset Boulevard, three blocks inland from Pacific Coast Highway. Open Tuesday–Sunday, 9 A.M.–4:45 P.M. (occasionally closed on Saturdays; call ahead to make sure); temple open Tuesday–Sunday, 1–4:45 P.M. Admission: free. Phone: (213) 454-4114.

It might be hard to imagine now, but in the 1920s and 1930s California's most charismatic religious leader was an Indian guru named Yogananda. He founded a series of shrines and temples, and this is the most striking one of all. A small lake surrounded by wooded paths takes up most of the grounds. A very non-Indian windmill houses the prayer temple, and a 1950s-style white houseboat (Yogananda's private retreat) floats in the water. The Golden Lotus Archway is a huge white gate topped with an eight-foot-tall gold-plated lotus bud. Behind the archway lies a shrine containing some of Mahatma Gandhi's ashes. On the west side of the lake is the gift shop and Yogananda Museum (open Tuesday–Sunday, 11 A.M.–4 P.M.).

PALOS VERDES ESTATES
(South of Redondo Beach)

Malaga Cove Fountain: in the parking lot in front of the Malaga Cove Mall, near the intersection of Via Campesina and Via Corta. Visible anytime.

This shameless fountain features four comely mermaids holding their breasts and smiling demurely as water spurts furiously out of their nipples. Shield your children's eyes!

PASADENA

Doo Dah Parade: the Sunday following Thanksgiving, noon–2 P.M. Parade starts at Fair Oaks and Union, goes north on Fair Oaks to Holly, east on Holly to Raymond, south on Raymond to Colorado, west on Colorado to Pasadena, south on Pasadena to Green, east on Green to Fair Oaks, and south on Fair Oaks to oblivion. For more information, call (818) 796-2591.

This satirical extravaganza began as a parody of Pasadena's Rose Parade but has since taken on a life of its own and has become nearly as famous. The main rule is, anyone who follows rules has no place in the parade. Every year the parade is different, so how can we describe it? Expect police officers in drag, floats made of beer cans, precision nose-picking teams, and a mockery of every conceivable parade cliché. No single event sums up "the California experience" better than this one.

SAN JUAN CAPISTRANO

The Swallows' Return: March 19. Mission San Juan Capistrano, 3182 Camino Capistrano, at Spring Street. For more information, call (714) 493-1424.

Every year, for over two centuries, hordes of swallows have been coming back to Capistrano, and always on the same day. They come to the mission from Argentina, a staggering 6,000 miles away, to nest and raise their young. Local celebrations mark the birds' annual arrival, as well as their departure—which is always on October 23.

SAN PEDRO

Blessing of the Fleet: the Sunday nearest the full moon in late September or early October, 10 A.M.–noon. Fishing-boat marina adjacent to Ports O' Call Village (south end of Harbor Boulevard). For more information, call (213) 832-7272.

San Pedro is Los Angeles' harbor (though many Angelenos don't even know they *have* a harbor). The fishing fleet is much beloved here. As part of the annual Fishermen's Fiesta, the cardinal of Los Angeles rides in a boat among the boats of the fishermen. He sprinkles holy water on the fleet and pronounces prayers for its safety.

Whale Fiesta: first Saturday in June, 9 A.M.–4:30 P.M. Activities are centered around the Cabrillo Marine

Museum, 3720 Stephen White Drive (south of downtown) and on Cabrillo Beach directly across from the museum. For more information, call (213) 548-7563.

Every year, museum staff members select a different breed of whale for festival-goers to build out of sand. They build the whale life-size, which makes for one of the world's largest sand sculptures. A helicopter flies overhead at 2 P.M. to take aerial photos of the granular leviathan. Volunteers stay at the beach overnight, keeping the beast company and guarding it from would-be Ahabs.

SANTA MONICA

Camera Obscura: inside the senior center, Palisades Park, 1450 Ocean Avenue, at Broadway. Open Monday–Friday, 9 A.M.–4 P.M.; Saturday–Sunday, 11 A.M.–4 P.M. Admission: free. Phone: (213) 393-7593. Ask at front desk for camera obscura info sheet.

Get a whole different view of Santa Monica's bay and pier via this Newtonian miracle. A mile of scenery is projected on a big platform; the effect is like that of watching a film projected on a screen, except what you're watching here is real.

Singing Beach Chairs: on the beach, across from the Sea Castle apartment building, whose address is 1725 Promenade. Visible anytime. Admission: free. For more information, call (213) 458-8350.

Two giant turquoise-green chairs perch on the sand, lifeguard style. They were made for this beach, and made to sing: A series of pipes along the chairs' backs catches the wind and produces a soulful, wavering music that sounds part panpipe, part oboe, and almost human. The music can be heard only on or near the 14-foot-high chairs, so climb up (each one has room enough for two), tune in, and zone out.

STUDIO CITY

The Retake Room: 3953 Laurel Grove Avenue, just off Ventura Boulevard. Open Monday–Saturday 11 A.M.–5 P.M. Phone: (818) 508-7762.

You never buy things second-hand, huh? Not good enough for you, huh? This shop sells the castoffs of the stars. When the big studios' wardrobe departments clean

MINIATURE GOLF

We like funny buildings. We don't care what they're used for (if anything), just as long as they're in a ridiculous shape. And there's no better place to find crazy architecture in heavy doses than at miniature golf courses. Here are three of the L.A. area's best.

ANAHEIM

<u>Camelot Golfland:</u> 3200 East Carpenter Avenue, near the corner of La Palma Avenue and Kramer Boulevard. Open Monday–Thursday, 10 A.M.–11 P.M.; Friday–Sunday, 10 A.M.–midnight. Admission: $4.25; children under 12, $3.25 (per 18 holes played). Phone: (714) 630-3340.

This isn't a miniature golf course: It's a miniature golf empire. Five 18-hole courses feature more than their fair share of pint-sized architectural follies. The theme is medieval, somewhat: A fairy-tale castle has a drawbridge and a moat. Two lifeless suits of armor fail to do battle with intruding dragons. Fountains, ponds, and a well provide aquatic distraction, whereas the less wealthy holes have to make do with humble but quaint cottages.

<u>Golf 'n' Stuff:</u> 1656 South Harbor Boulevard, near Katella. Open daily, 9 A.M.–midnight. Admission: $4.50; children 6–12, $3.50; children under 6, free. Phone: (714) 778-4100.

A Chinese temple, pots of gold, castles and drawbridges, airplanes, windmills, a miniature schoolhouse, and plenty of loop-de-loops make this one of the most diverse 36-hole courses around.

REDONDO BEACH

<u>Malibu Castle Park Golf:</u> 2410 West Compton Boulevard. Open Monday–Thursday, 11 A.M.–11 P.M.; Friday, 11 A.M.–midnight; Saturday, 10 A.M.–midnight; Sunday, 10 A.M.–11 P.M. Admission: $4.50; children 13 and under, $3.50. Phone: (213) 643-5166 or (213) 643-5167.

Thirty-six holes of top-flight wackiness: a huge skull with water squirting out of it; a Taj Mahal; a pirate ship with towering masts and threatening cannons; and the usual assortment of windmills, bridges, and lopsided houses.

their closets, the results end up here. Does *that* make you change your tune?

VAN NUYS

Tower of Wooden Pallets: 15357 Magnolia Boulevard, on the sliver of land between Sepulveda Boulevard and the San Diego Freeway. (Technically the tower is within Van Nuys city limits, but this neighborhood is generally thought of as part of Sherman Oaks.) Open daily, 9 A.M.– dusk. Admission: free. Phone: (818) 784-5541.

In 1951, Daniel Van Meter somewhat unwittingly acquired ten truckloads of wooden pallets from the Schlitz Brewery. The building-block instinct took over, and Van Meter started stacking 2,000 of the pallets on top of each other until he had created his masterpiece. The vaguely conical Tower of Wooden Pallets is about 30 feet across at the base, and tapers to 10 feet across at its nearly 25-foot summit. Van Meter welcomes visitors to his debris-filled, two-acre backyard. You might want to call ahead and make sure he's home, but even if he's out to lunch he says he doesn't mind interested people coming in to take a gander.

VERNON

Farmer John Pig Murals: on the walls of the meat-packing facility, on East Vernon Avenue, Soto Street, and Bandini Street. Visible anytime. Phone: (213) 583-4621.

You know what they say about meat-packing plants: that they're deathmongers; that they smell. Thirty years ago the Farmer John patriarch, sick and tired of this bad rap, commissioned a Hollywood scene painter to cover the walls of his buildings with funny animal murals. Today you can drive by and see jolly, almost-human pigs cavorting in the mud, rolling in the grass, being taken for walks by the farmer's daughter. The original artist fell off a scaffold while painting these and died. (Sausages' revenge?) But he did such a good job making these porkers look rebellious that you'll end up loving pigs— and hating bacon.

WATTS

Watts Towers: 1727 East 107th Street, Watts (which is technically part of the city of Los Angeles), east of

Central Avenue. Visible from the sidewalk anytime; close-up tours not available until 1992. Admission: free. For more information, call the Watts Towers Art Center at (213) 732-1243.

This is it, the original urban eccentric folk art, built by Simon Rodia over a three-decade span. They've finally gotten the respect they deserved, having survived wrecking balls, riots, and apathy. Now safely enshrined as a national landmark, the towers are being spruced up for a public reopening in 1992. In the meantime, you can see from a distance the 100-foot-tall spindly spires made of cement, shells, and garbage. You can still inspect close-up the often-overlooked walls, which Rodia built in the same spirit as the towers and out of the same materials. Intimidate your arty friends by saying, "Oh, I've just come back from visiting the Watts *walls.*"

WEST HOLLYWOOD

Tail O' The Pup: 329 San Vicente Boulevard, at Beverly Boulevard, next to Fidelity Federal Savings, kittycorner from the Hard Rock Café. Open daily, 6 A.M.–8:30 P.M. Phone: (213) 652-4517.

To many people, this giant weenie symbolizes L.A. It has been around as long as anyone can remember: a hot dog stand in the shape of a huge hot dog, architectural souvenir of a more interesting time, complete with mustard, bun, and striped awning. Employees call it "The Tail."

WOODLAND HILLS
(San Fernando Valley)

John Ehn's Old Trapper's Lodge: on the grounds of Pierce College, 6201 Winnetka Avenue. Sculptures are on the west side of campus in an area called Cleveland Park, next to Warner Center. Visible anytime. Admission: free. For more information, call (818) 719-6400.

John Ehn, who actually was a trapper at one point in his life, built a motel in Sun Valley in 1941 and started making cement statues to decorate it. He got the inspiration while watching an artist do his portrait. His statues seized control of the yard: a 14-foot-high kidnap scene; life-size, pensive dance-hall girls with his daughters' faces; a hilarious fake cemetery whose epitaphs reached new heights of honesty and crudity. Ehn affixed western

and pioneer relics to walls, trees, and fences. Old
Trapper's Lodge, the by-now-legendary folk art motel,
faced possible destruction in 1988 when the late John
Ehn's children were forced to sell the motel to
developers. In the nick of time, Pierce College offered to
install the outdoor art on its campus; so now this con-
troversial life-work is again safe and sound in a new location. Pierce College may lack the charm of the old motel,
but it's better than oblivion.

THE CENTRAL COAST

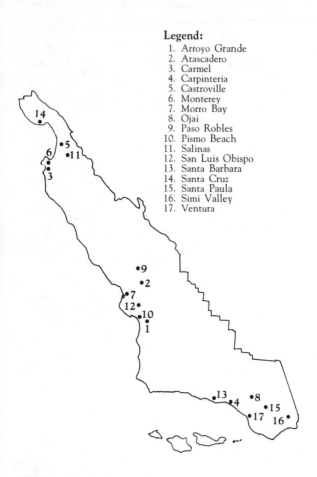

Legend:
1. Arroyo Grande
2. Atascadero
3. Carmel
4. Carpinteria
5. Castroville
6. Monterey
7. Morro Bay
8. Ojai
9. Paso Robles
10. Pismo Beach
11. Salinas
12. San Luis Obispo
13. Santa Barbara
14. Santa Cruz
15. Santa Paula
16. Simi Valley
17. Ventura

The coast north of San Francisco is too cold and windy. The beaches around Los Angeles and the south are too hot, crowded, and over-developed. The truly idyllic California coast, the coast of your dreams, lies *between* the state's two big urban areas, yet remains strangely ignored by both of them. For better or worse, the central coast continues at its own pace, cultivating its own idiosyncracies unencumbered by outside influences, bad weather, or the need to maintain an acceptable appearance. An artichoke festival? Give it a go! A monument to a car crash? Why the hell not? A theme hotel based on the words of an absurdist poem? Who's gonna complain?

ATASCADERO

Mudhole Follies: third weekend in October. Most activities take place in the Sunken Gardens, in front of the E. G. Lewis Building. Events listed here begin Saturday, around noon. For more information, call (805) 466-4931.

Atascadero means "mudhole" in Spanish, so there really should be mud wrestling at this festival. But there isn't. Instead, local bigwigs compete in a bathtub race, in which roller skates are attached to plastic tubs with people in them...and a centipede race, in which five people share a single pair of ten-foot-long skis...and giant inner-tube rolling. What reaction would this get from Edward Garner Lewis, who founded Atascadero in 1913 as a model community, and who ended up in jail for mail fraud?

CAMBRIA
(22 miles northwest of Morro Bay)

Nitwit Ridge: on Hillcrest Drive, one block up from Main Street. Visible anytime. Admission: free. For more information, call (805) 927-3624.

Art Beal, who used to call himself Captain Nitwit or Dr. Tinkerpaw, will occasionally toddle out onto the balcony of the dilapidated vision of madness he calls home to hurl invectives at the universe and urinate on unfortunate passersby. We're not saying Beal hasn't built the most quirky, outlandish house on the west coast; it's just that he's become somewhat unbalanced in the process. Nitwit Ridge, aka Dr. Tinkerpaw's Castle, has nine levels; undulating walls; and towers of cemented-together rocks, metal, TVs, toilets, and junk. It took Beal 60 years to complete the house. Now it's disintegrating, yet Beal refuses to cooperate with anyone who wants to fix it up. Why not? It's *his* house, and he can do what he wants, despite what meddlesome do-gooders may think. Just don't stand under the balcony.

CAPITOLA

Sand Castle Contest: the Sunday before Labor Day, on Capitola Beach. Registration begins at 8 A.M.; judging begins at 1:30 P.M. For more information, call (408) 462-3419.

This is part of the Begonia Festival, a decades-old tradition in Capitola. There's more than enough sand to go around as locals and out-of-towners head for the beach, dreaming of sandy victory.

CARMEL

Sand Castle Contest: third Saturday in October. Judging takes place in early afternoon, on the beach. For more information, call (408) 624-2522.

Thousands turn up every year to watch the builders at work. Each year, a different theme dominates the contest, which is the brainchild of the American Institute of Architects—who know more about castles than the rest of us.

Una Jeffers' Unicorn Collection: at Tor House, on Carmel Point, just south of Carmel. House is bounded by Ocean View Avenue and Stewart Way. Tours given Friday–Saturday, 10 A.M.–3 P.M. Admission: $3.50; high school students, $1.50. No children under 12 allowed on tour. Reservations required. Phone: (408) 624-1813.

Robinson Jeffers, who built this stunning house, was a famous poet. Una Jeffers, for whom he built the house, was a famous poet's wife. Unicorns were her personal mascot, and through the hour-long tour you can see about a hundred of them. Keep your eyes peeled and you'll see unicorns in paintings, miniatures, carvings, china figurines...everything but the real thing.

CARPINTERIA

Santa Claus, CA: on Highway 101, three miles north of Carpinteria, on the west side of the road. Visible anytime. For more information, call (805) 684-3515.

Who's that big hitchhiker in the red suit? You know darn well who it is. It's Santa, standing guard over the town named in his honor. Tiny, unincorporated Santa

Claus, California, is a toy shop, a Mexican restaurant, a date-shake parlor, and little else, but still.... An elephantine Frosty the Snowman keeps Santa company up on the roof, and postcards mailed from the toy shop get a "Santa Claus, California" postmark—even in July. At press time, devilish plans were underway to replace the town's old red-and-white motif with a blue-and-beige "New England Seaport" theme: thus proving that, whether or not there is a Santa, there most definitely is not a God.

CASTROVILLE

Artichoke Festival: third weekend in September. Events take place at various locations and times. Artichoke Queen coronation: Friday, 10 P.M., Castroville Community Center. Recipe contest: Saturday, 9 A.M.– noon, North County High School. Artichoke eating contest: Saturday, 2 P.M., Community Center. Artichoke parade: Sunday, 10 A.M., Merritt Street. For more information, call (408) 633-2465.

An artichoke is the only food that takes up more space *after* it has been eaten. The unruly pile of nibbled leaves inevitably has twice the volume of the compact artichoke it came from. When the "Artichoke Capitol of the World" holds its annual shindig, a high point is the artichoke eating contest: A recent winner managed to eat over a pound of pure artichoke meat (i.e., his pile of leaves weighed one pound less than the artichokes they came from). The recipe contest ranges from Artichokes Prosciutto to Clam-Stuffed Artichokes. And you've never seen anyone quite as silly as the people in the parade dressed up in artichoke outfits.

Giant Artichoke Restaurant: 11261 Merritt Street, next to Highway 156. Open daily, 6:30 A.M.–8 P.M. Phone: (408) 633-3204.

"Hey—they *do* grow big artichokes around here, don't they?" No, no—that's a cement artichoke, ten feet of greenish-gray realism. The edible artichokes are inside the restaurant, where the chefs of this possibly unique artichoke-themed eatery serve up at least eight different recipes based on the tasty thistle. Artichoke quiche, soup, cake; steamed, sautéed and fried artichokes. If you lost all your teeth in a bowling accident last October, don't waste your time coming here.

BUTTERFLY TREES

Every year, swarms of Monarch butterflies migrate to California's central coast, attracted by the mild winter climate. Some unfathomable directional sense guides them to the exact same trees every year, even though different butterflies return each time. The butterflies blanket the trees, and sturdy branches bend under their weight. The city of Pacific Grove has made a career out of publicizing its butterfly trees; few people realize that Pacific Grove is only one of many resorts on the Butterfly Riviera. Here's a list of the central coast's *other* butterfly wintering grounds, from north to south down the coast.

Santa Cruz: in Natural Bridges State Beach, at the far western edge of town, at the end of West Cliff Drive and Delaware Avenue; main area is the eucalyptus grove around the visitors' center. Phone: (408) 423-4609.

The butterflies arrive in October, fill the trees by December, and leave in February.

Pacific Grove: on the grounds of the Butterfly Grove Inn, at 1073 Lighthouse Avenue, in the eucalyptus and pine groves, near Ridge Road; also in George Washington Park, bordered by Melrose, Short, and Alder Streets, and Sinex Avenue, just south of the other grove. Phone: (408) 373-4921.

Early arrivals show up in late October or early November; they're gone by the beginning of March.

Morro Bay: south of town in the picnic area off State Park Road. Look for the part of the picnic grounds that borders on the golf course, especially the area around campsites 114 and 118, south of Park View Drive. Preferred trees are pine and eucalyptus. Phone: (805) 772-7434.

Best time to view the butterflies here is from November to January.

Pismo Beach: in the area just south of Pismo Beach, between Highway 1 and the beach, adjacent to Grover City, in the eucalyptus and Monterey pine groves. Phone: (800) 443-7778.

Here they come again, those purty-lookin' six-legged critters. Check 'em out November through March.

CHOLAME
(25 miles east of Paso Robles)

James Dean's Death Site and Memorial: right in front of the Cholame Post Office, on the north side of Highway 46, east of Maggie's Café; look for a metal monument around a tree. Cholame is about one mile southwest of where Highways 41 and 46 meet. For more information, call the post office at (805) 238-1390 or Maggie's at (805) 238-5652.

James Dean's career started East of Eden but ended here, east of Paso Robles. This is where, on that fateful date, 9–30-55, Jimmy's Porsche decelerated from 100 mph to 0 mph in less than a second, sending Jimmy to that big ranch house/planetarium in the sky. The memorial, made of brass, aluminum, and steel, is set on a cement block and has a smarmy inscription. Oddly, Dean's death is only one of several disasters to strike the mysterious and tiny "town" (just a wide place in the road) of Cholame, which, by the way, is pronounced sha-LAM. In 1975 the town was struck by a meteor shower, an event that all the locals claim never happened; and the whole area is constantly barraged by earthquakes, lying as it does directly on the San Andreas Fault. Bad vibes, man, bad vibes.

HALCYON
(One mile south of Arroyo Grande)

Temple of the People and Halcyon Cemetery: Temple is at 906 South Halcyon Road at Temple Drive, west side of the road; cemetery is three blocks west on The Pike near the intersection of Elm Street. Both are visible anytime. Phone (the Temple): (805) 489-2822.

Modern-day religious Utopias, such as Jonestown and Rajneeshpuram, have soured public opinion of idealistic communities founded by eccentric spiritual leaders. Halcyon is just about the only one of California's many visionary religious colonies that still stands and remains true to its principles. Today Halcyon is just a few blocks and some farmland—but it does have the Temple of the People, meeting place and spiritual headquarters of the 36th Order of Wisdom, the religious sect that founded and still supports Halcyon. The temple has three curving sides, a triangular roof, columns, and a spiffy blue-and-white paint job. This is one of those "every-architectural-detail-has-religious-significance"-type places. Down the street is the creepy-crawly Halcyon Cemetery, sporting a spiked metal fence and a creaking gate.

MONTEREY

Glass-Bottom Boat Harbor Tours: Wharf #1 (right side). Tours depart every half-hour, Monday–Friday, noon–4 P.M. (closing time depends on the amount of business that day); Saturday and Sunday, 11 A.M.–4 P.M. (approximately). Admission: $2.50. Phone: (408) 372-7150.

Won't King Neptune be angry when he sees you peering down into his private domain through a panel of glass! Every tour is different because the ocean is always different; the boat is like a traveling aquarium. Glass-bottom boaters commonly see otters and sea lions on the tour, but the possibilities are endless. Great white shark? Mermaid? Beer can? Who can say?

The Jabberwock Bed and Breakfast: 598 Laine Street, at Hoffman Avenue, four blocks from Cannery Row. Room rates: $82–$115. Phone: (408) 372-4777.

The next time Alice and the Mad Hatter sneak off for a tryst in Monterey, this is where they're gonna stay. Guest rooms have names you'll remember from the poem: The Brillig, The Toves, The Mimsy, etc. (Cheapest room is the Tulgey Wood.) The clocks here run backward; the proprietors tuck you in at night with cookies and milk; there's a White Rabbit on the premises. The Walrus and the Carpenter would relish the breakfast menu, which features snarkleberry flumpsious, razzleberry flabjous, and burndt blumbleberry. Gotta make a phone call? Head for the Burbling Room. A snack? The Tum-Tum Room, of course. Remember: Giring and gimbling are strictly out-grabe.

Santa Rosalia Fleet Blessing: the first Sunday after Labor Day, 11 A.M. Procession begins at San Carlos Cathedral (on Church Street); continues down Alvarado Street to the Custom House Plaza and Wharf #1. For more information, call (408) 373-8451.

A life-size statue of Santa Rosalia journeys down to the sea on a float and, later, is held aloft on fishermen's shoulders. It's a ritual that was born in Palermo, Sicily. On the wharf, the bishop bestows blessings as fishing boats chug back and forth around him. Finally, a wreath is thrown into the sea in memory of those Monterey fishermen who never came home.

MOORPARK
(Eight miles west of Simi Valley)

Zoo School's Animal Shows: Exotic Animal Training and Management Department, Moorpark College, 7075 Campus Road, just east of town, off Highway 118. "Zoo" is at bottom edge of campus. Shows every Sunday, 3 P.M. Admission: $2; children, $1. Phone: (805) 529-2321.

At the only college in America where you can learn to

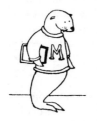

teach sea lions to jump through hoops, students show off their knowledge in weekly extravaganzas. Cavorting at the shows are some of the school's 300 talented animals: baboons, llamas, parrots, sea lions, and more. Students who graduate from here get jobs training animals for theme parks and the movies.

MORRO BAY

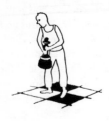

Giant Chessboard: on Embarcadero and Front Streets, at the foot of the "Centennial Stairway" leading down from Morro Bay Boulevard. Pieces available daily, 8 A.M.–5 P.M. Call the Parks and Recreation Department at (805) 772-1214, ext. 226, to get access to the pieces.

Build those biceps and develop those deltoids with an athletic, sweaty game of...chess? Morro Bay's giant outdoor chess set, inspired by Europe's outdoor sets, has pieces that weigh up to thirty pounds each. The city fathers claim that during a typical game a player will lift around 1,000 pounds; but if you include carrying the pieces off the board after captures, the estimate should be closer to 2,000 pounds. Who says chess is for wimps?

OJAI

Gallery of Historical Figurines: at the intersection of McNell Road and Reeves Road, about four miles east of the center of town. Open Saturday and Sunday, 1–5 P.M.; presentations on Saturday evenings once a month or so; call for dates and to make reservations. Admission: $1; children under 12, free; presentations cost $5 per person. Phone: (805) 646-6339.

Don't call 'em dolls, whatever you do. George Stuart—historian, monologuist, and creator of these quarter-life-size figurines—would (quite rightfully) take offense. He painstakingly researches the historical background for each model, so that the final product is not only chock full of details but also chock full of the *right* details. Are the Oscar Wilde figure's cufflinks the same kind that the real Oscar Wilde wore? Are Peter the Great's epaulets just right? Is that cowboy wearing his spurs right side up? You can bet they are. On occasional Saturdays, Stuart holds 90-minute salons, during which he expounds upon matters historical, as represented by his beloved dolls—*oops*.

PISMO BEACH

Sand Castle Contest and Clam Dig: second Saturday in October, on the beach, near the pier. For more information, call (805) 773-4658 or (800) 443-7778.

Castles emerge from the sand as, nearby, hopefuls dig for treasure. Pismo clamshells, each marked with a number, lie buried in the sand. If you find one, you can use it to claim a prize that has a matching code number. Now that the actual Pismo clam has been almost dug out of existence, a treasure hunt is the next best thing.

SALINAS

Hat in Three Stages of Landing: in Sherwood Park, 940 North Main, behind the Community Center. Always visible. Phone: (408) 758-7351.

The Jolly Green Giant, having fallen on hard times and taken a job harvesting lettuce in the Salinas Valley, attends the Salinas Rodeo one day and throws his hat off with joy when his buddy Li'l Sprout wins the calf-roping competition. His gigantic straw hat sails through the air and lands gently in the field behind the nearby Community Center. It was perhaps this image that artist Claes Oldenburg had in mind when he designed "Hat in Three Stages of Landing." Three versions of the same vast metal "straw" hat slowly descend to ground level. It is, in a phrase, surrealistically mundane.

SAN LUIS OBISPO

Bubblegum Alley: between 733 and 737 Higuera Street on the south side of the street, between Broad and Garden Streets; the alley extends one-half block and connects to a parking lot on Marin Street. Always open. Admission: free.

Bubblegum Alley is not a quaint row of candy and toy stores. Nor is it an official city landmark. No, Bubblegum Alley is a disgusting narrow passageway whose walls are covered with years and years' worth of multicolored, premasticated blobs of bubblegum. Generations of youngsters have taken their drool-lubricated mouthfuls of Raspberry Dubble Bubble and, with it, spelled out their initials or the date or such inspirational messages as "Get Naked" and "21 Bun Salute." The chaotic, sticky masterpiece fairly begs for you to go buy a couple of packs of Bazooka Joe and add your own personal touch.

Madonna Inn: 100 Madonna Road, at the southern end of town, just west of Highway 101. Room rates: $76–$180. Phone: (805) 543-3000.

Despite what the name may lead you to believe, this is *not* the place that turned Mary away when she was having labor pains. This one was built 1,958 years later, which is as convincing an alibi as we've ever heard. Each of its 109 guest rooms has a different theme. The Caveman Room is made of rocks and has a waterfall shower. The Old Mill Room has a functioning mill inside. The Austrian Room is pure elegant Hapsburg blue. And don't forget the Safari Room; the Daisy Mae Room; and plenty of red, pink, and heart-shaped honeymoon suites. Downstairs, the legendary men's room has a rock waterfall urinal activated when your wee-wee breaks the photoelectric beam.

Motel Inn: 2223 Monterey Street, at the north end of town next to Highway 101. Room rates: $30 and up. Phone: (805) 543-4000.

Back in the 1920s, when Los Angeles first emerged as a place worth driving to, there was no Highway 5; just winding old Highway 101, on which the cars of the day were lucky to do 40 mph. The trip from San Francisco to L.A. took *two* days, which meant you had to spend the night somewhere in the middle. What's in the middle? Why, San Luis Obispo, of course. In 1926, clairvoyant entrepreneur Arthur Heineman got the idea for a "motor hotel" where both cars and their drivers could rest for a night. But "motor hotel" was too cumbersome, so he combined the words to make "motel," unknowingly coining a word that by now is part of 150 languages worldwide. The undisputed first motel still thrives today, featuring quaint mission-style architecture and U-pick tangerine trees.

Renaissance Faire: a weekend in late June (varies). At El Chorro Regional Park, six miles northwest of town on Highway 1. Park is across the highway from Cuesta College. Faire is open Saturday, 10 A.M.–6 P.M.; Sunday, 10 A.M.–5 P.M. Admission: $5; seniors and children 6–12, $3; children under 6, free. For more information, call (805) 549-9260 or (805) 543-1323.

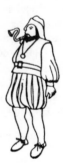

It's 1565, and the Virgin Queen presides over her subjects: courtiers, peasants, pirates, pipers, acrobats, gypsies, swordsmen, and hundreds of other costumed Renaissance characters who play their roles with loving care and doggedly insist on speaking in funny accents. Three stages feature jugglers, puppet shows, and raucous Shakespeare playlets. If you can't afford the Agoura Hills RenFaire (and who can, on a 16th-century budget?), you'll find this one a satisfyingly cozy affair. But hey, if this is 1565, where are the Chumash Indians?

SAN MIGUEL ISLAND
(28 miles off the Santa Barbara coast)

Cast Forest and Ranch Remnants: Trips to the island are conducted by Island Packers, 1867 Spinnaker Drive, Ventura, at the harbor. Trips usually leave once a month from May to October; dates change each year. One-day trips last from 7 A.M. to 6 P.M., and cost $60, $50 for children; two-day overnight trips to San Miguel and Santa Rosa Islands cost $170, $150 for children. For more information about excursions and to make reservations, call Island Packers at (805) 642-7688 or (805) 642-1393; for more information on San Miguel Island itself, call Channel Islands National Park at (805) 644-8262.

The only remains of this windy, desolate island's once-flourishing forest is the Caliche Forest. Calcium carbonate sand particles, whipped up by the incessant winds, embedded themselves in the crevices of dead and dying tree trunks; the wood absorbed the minerals, and eventually the trees became totally calcified. The spooky white stumps and branches are sometimes called the Ghost Forest. Also here is the foundation of Rancho Rambouillet, former home of Herbert Lester, self-declared "King of San Miguel." The strangely shaped house, built of wood salvaged from shipwrecks, burned down a few years ago, but the ranger's telling of Lester's eccentric story will more than make up for the missing boards. San Miguel is also home to a large seal and sea lion rookery, unexploded WWII bombs, and—somewhere—Juan Cabrillo's unmarked grave.

SANTA BARBARA

Sand Castle Contest: first Sunday in August. On East Beach, next to Cabrillo Avenue, about one mile east of the pier, near the zoo. Construction begins at noon; judging begins at 3 P.M. For more information, call (805) 966-6110.

Contestants get a 20-foot-by-20-foot plot of sand, and a scant three hours to build castles or sculptures. A special "Do Your Own Thing" category allows builders to adorn sand creations with water-soluble paint, feathers, shells, and seaweed.

Summer Solstice Celebration: The Saturday preceding solstice (June 21). Parade begins at noon on lower State Street, downtown. For more information, call (805) 965-3396.

Okay, so the Reagans live in Santa Barbara. But so do a lot of wacky nutballs who dress as Vikings, hammers, pizzas, and grapes and march through the center of town. Anything goes here (as long as it doesn't have a motor): Recent floats have included a wooden ship on wheels, a dragon, and a 25-foot whale. The scene is hallucinogenic, with lots of face paint, streamers, and large, clanking visual puns that hop up and down shouting, "Get it? Get it?"

SANTA CRUZ

The Last Supper in Wax: 526 Broadway, next to Ocean Street. Open daily, 10 A.M.–5 P.M. Admission: donation. Phone: (408) 426-5787.

Leonardo da Vinci gets a lot of credit for being a visionary genius. He thought the craftspeople of the future would be constructing full-sized corkscrew helicopters based on his drawing. Instead they've built a full-sized Last Supper based on his painting, which is probably the last thing he expected. Some visionary. Still, this is better than wearing 3-D glasses. The 13 wax figures are life-sized, totally true to the painting, and hyperrealistic. The mother-daughter team that slaved over the figures spent eight months just on the one task of putting in each hair individually.

The Mystery Spot: 1953 Branciforte Drive, north of town, east of Highway 17; once on Branciforte Drive, turn west on Mystery Spot Road (signs will guide you). Open daily, 9:30 A.M.–4:30 P.M. Admission: $3; children 5–11, $1.50. Phone: (408) 423-8897.

Pity all the poor debunkers of the world. They spend every waking hour crusading against what they call "pseudoscience," saving the world from its own ignorance and gullibility. Over and over again they've conclusively demonstrated that astrology is bogus, ghosts and UFOs are just wishful thinking, and mystery spots are about as authentic as the fight scenes in a kung fu movie. All to no avail. Proof and rationality are irrelevant to the average American. Science is *boring*—mystery spots are *interesting*. It's as simple as that. So don't expect the Mystery Spot to ever go begging for tourists. Where else can Bay Area visitors watch balls roll uphill, feel themselves changing height, and perceive with their very eyes what science says is impossible?

Surfing Museum: in the lighthouse, at Lighthouse Point on West Cliff Drive, west of downtown. Open in summer, Monday–Friday, noon–5 P.M.; Saturday, 10 A.M.–6 P.M.; in winter, daily, noon–5 P.M. Admission: free, but donations are welcomed. Phone: (408) 429-3429.

At this very moment, Gidget and Moondoggie are zooming up Highway 1 in their woody, on their way to this museum. They want to see the photos, boards, and other bitchin' artifacts that trace the sport from the 1930s to the 1980s. A special exhibit is devoted to surfing in Hawaii, then and now.

UCSC Slug Fest: a Friday afternoon in early October (date varies). In the parking lot at the corner of Cathcart Street and Pacific Avenue. for more information, call (408) 423-1111.

UCLA has its Bruins; UC Santa Cruz has its Slugs. Every year the town welcomes its university students with a blowout in honor of the school's mascot. Respect for the species forbids any slug racing, but on the scene are people in slug costumes, slug-related comedy acts, and food that *looks* like slugs but doesn't taste like them. Pastries are adorned with rampaging frosting slugs; long chocolate-chip cookies are banana-flavored—evoking the spotted banana slug. T-shirts on sale here depict the slow-moving slime wreakers in various attitudes of work and play.

SANTA PAULA

California Oil Museum: 1003 Main Street, at 10th Street. Open Wednesday–Sunday, 10 A.M.–4 P.M. Admission: free. Phone: (805) 525-6672.

A huge, carefully crafted, pre-1910 wooden oil derrick is the highlight of this museum, which was created to preserve obsolete oil-drilling equipment and lore. Many of these artifacts were literally dug up in old oilfields. Also here is a replica of a 1933 Union Oil service station, and plans are underway for a new electronic exhibit.

Santa Paula Dental Museum: 722 East Main Street, at 8th Street. Open: Tuesday–Thursday, 9 A.M.–noon and 2–6 P.M.; also sometimes open the same hours every other Saturday and every other Monday. Call ahead of time to make sure. Admission: free. Phone: (805) 525-3001.

One glance at this self-described "private hobby run amok" will keep you brushing and flossing from now 'til doomsday. Did you know the first dental drills were foot-powered by treadle mills? The one on display here will make you thank the Tooth Fairy that you live in the days of alternating current. Skull and tooth models and examples of crowns and bridges lend a macabre air to the whole collection. Best of all is an old book that illustrates the history of dentistry from the stone age to the present, a tale more horrifying than *The Shining* or the Old Testament.

SEASIDE
(Three miles east of Monterey)

Bed Race: second Sunday in September. Bed Parade is at 11 A.M., on Canyon Del Rey, from Francis Avenue to Sonoma Avenue. Races: 1–4 P.M., down Canyon Del Rey, starting at Harcourt Avenue, past the city park. For more information, call (408) 394-6501.

Competitors decorate their beds to look like missiles, insects, or the Trojan Horse. And speed is the least of their problems, as judges take into account the quality of the riders' costumes, craftsmanship, and talent for making the audience laugh. It's a safe race, too—most of the riders wear "bed belts" and helmets.

SIMI VALLEY

Grandma Prisbrey's Bottle Village: 4595 Cochran Street, near Highway 118. Never open, but always visible through the fence. Admission: free. For more information, call the Preserve Bottle Village Committee at (805) 583-1627.

Why can't we all have grandmas like Grandma Prisbrey? Not content to live in a trailer park or Leisure World, she spent nearly 30 years turning bottles, cement, tiles, car parts, and societal castoffs into Bottle Village. And it really is a village, with many houses and a main "street"—paved with tiles and, well, *stuff*. The buildings are mostly made, as you might expect, out of bottles, with their necks pointing out so the flat bottoms on the inside look like stained glass. Grandma Prisbrey is now well into her 90s and lives elsewhere, so Bottle Village is officially closed to the public as volunteers figure out how to restore it. Meanwhile, you'll have to be content with taking pictures from behind the fence.

SOLVANG
(28 miles northwest of Santa Barbara)

Danish Days: third weekend in September. Activities take place all over town. For more information, call (805) 688-6144.

Solvang is a Danish town—in that dreamlike, half-real California way. Fake storks nest on the pertly peaked rooftops; windmill imagery is a bit overobvious; we are selling typical Danish souvenirs, don't ya know. The only thing missing is Danny Kaye. Danish Days rubs it in— with parades, *aebelskiver*, performers, and dancing in the street.

Viking Ship in a Church: Bethania Lutheran Church, 603 Atterdag Road, at Laurel. Open daily, 10 A.M.–5 P.M. Admission: free. Phone: (805) 688-4637.

The church itself, patterned after a Danish country church, has handsome wooden fixtures, a 1,000-pipe organ, and occasional services held in Danish. In honor of Denmark's seafaring heritage, it's also got an elaborate Viking ship hanging from the ceiling—not quite life-size but still convincing. The Lutherans may have never claimed the Vikings' pagan souls, but they still managed to nab their ship.

VENTURA

Beatrice Wyatt's Yard: 223 South Olive Street, at the western end of Ventura, underneath the freeway next to the County Fairgrounds and railroad tracks. Always visible.

In a world where people take beautiful things and make them ugly, Beatrice Wyatt takes ugly things and makes them...well, maybe not beautiful exactly, but at least interesting. Towers of soft-drink cups, all salvaged from the garbage, lean at precarious angles. Her driveway has wall-to-wall carpeting made of discarded rug remnants. She meticulously paints stones and pinecones and places them purposely all around her property. Wyatt uses materials for her works that even the most trendy art student would blanch at the thought of: misshapen chunks of styrofoam, broken furniture, food containers. Two decades of collecting and composing have made Wyatt's yard into a riotous rebellion against the acceptable. Not only that, she likes getting visitors, too.

Golf 'n' Stuff Miniature Golf Course: 5555 Walker Street, next to Victoria Avenue in the Montalvo district of Ventura; Walker Street is parallel to and just north of Highway 101. Open Sunday–Thursday, 10 A.M.–midnight; Friday and Saturday, 10 A.M.–1 A.M. Admission: $4.50; children under five, free. Phone: (805) 644-7132.

Thirty-six holes of fantasy architecture include a pseudo-Kremlin, a gold mine, a humungous clock, a windmill, a castle, and plenty of waterfalls and palm trees. Just like home, ain't it?

The Windmill King: 93 North Ann Street, at Poli Street. From Highway 101, take the Main Street exit. Open daily, daylight hours. Phone: (805) 643-2449.

James Giminiani, the Windmill King, lives in a forest of giant candy-colored pinwheels. For years, he's been designing and crafting the wheels out of pine and redwood, painting them brightly, and arranging them in his yard. Most are for sale. And most hypnotic are the double- and triple-decker inventions, in which wheels spin simultaneously in opposite directions. As a child in Italy, 70 years ago, Giminiani helped his farmer father make waterwheels—he painted *those* bright colors, too—but now he mills wind instead of water. "Wind," he reasons, "is free to all."

THE CENTRAL VALLEY AND THE GOLD COUNTRY

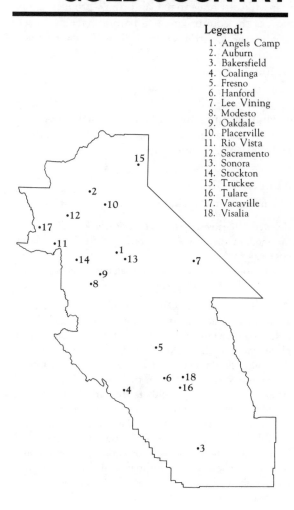

Legend:
1. Angels Camp
2. Auburn
3. Bakersfield
4. Coalinga
5. Fresno
6. Hanford
7. Lee Vining
8. Modesto
9. Oakdale
10. Placerville
11. Rio Vista
12. Sacramento
13. Sonora
14. Stockton
15. Truckee
16. Tulare
17. Vacaville
18. Visalia

This is the *real* California, the area that gave birth to the state and made it the economic superpower it is today. California might well still be part of Mexico (and a poor part at that), were it not for the discovery of gold in the Sierra foothills; San Francisco would be an abandoned mission on a windblown peninsula. And once the rush was over and most of the gold was played out, it was the development of agriculture in the valley that brought real prosperity. Though urban Californians like to brag that California's produce feeds most of the country, many urbanites have never set foot in the Central Valley. ("I don't want to get something on my shoe.") That's alright, say the Central Californians to the city slickers. You need us more than we need you.

Meanwhile, descendants of the '49ers have given up panning for gold and now make their fortunes running bed and breakfast hotels, ski resorts, and thermometer museums.

ALLENSWORTH
(45 miles north of Bakersfield)

Colonel Allensworth State Historic Park: adjacent to the modern town of Allensworth, on the west side of Highway 43. Visitors' Center is open daily, 8 A.M.–5 P.M., to give tours, but the park itself is always open. Admission: free. Phone: (805) 849-3433.

Years before Marcus Garvey sounded his call for an autonomous black nation, little-known Colonel Allen Allensworth, a former slave, founded this community as a place where blacks could live and work without having to endure discrimination. It is the only black Utopian community ever attempted in this country. The town of Allensworth lasted from 1908 to the early 1940s, though it had been dying for years because of an unforeseen drop in the water supply. In its heyday, Allensworth was a small but thriving all-black agricultural and intellectual community. The Department of Parks has now restored part of the ghost town and shows a film at the Visitors' Center about the town's history. This is a must-see on any tour of unusual ghost towns.

ANGELS CAMP
(15 miles northwest of Sonora)

Calaveras County Fair and Jumping Frog Jubilee: third weekend in May. Calaveras County Fairgrounds, just south of town along Highway 49. Frog jumping; Friday afternoon, all day Saturday, and all day Sunday; championship is on Sunday at 4 P.M. Admission per day: $5–$8; children, $3.50–$6.50. To enter or rent a frog: $3. Phone: (209) 736-2561.

When Samuel Clemens sat in his Mother Lode cabin, scribbling down a funny story he'd heard that day about a frog-jumping contest, he had no idea that 125 years later, tens of thousands of people would descend on that same town to hold frog-jumping contests in honor of his story. Yes, Sam, it's true. And anyone caught sneaking buckshot into the Jubilee will be tarred and feathered and run out of town.

AUBURN

The Dentist's Sculptures: 391 Auburn Ravine Road, between Elm and Palm, northern edge of town. Office is open Monday–Friday, 8 A.M.–5 P.M., but outdoor sculptures are visible anytime. Phone: (916) 885-2769.

Who *says* dentists can't sculpt 30-foot Amazonian Indians out of concrete and place them, Statue-of-Liberty-like, in front of their offices? Dr. Ken Fox started his project several decades ago, and his sculpting has in no way interfered with his drilling. A bow-and-arrow-wielding Indian in floor-length, flowing loincloth is only one of four towering outdoor statues; some smaller specimens reside in a gallery inside the office. Amazon Indians—in the Mother Lode? Says an associate of Dr. Fox: "He likes Amazon Indians."

BAKERSFIELD

Deschwanden's Shoe Repairing: 931 Chester Street (at 10th). Visible anytime. Phone: (805) 324-7292.

It seems Prince Charming found this big shoe after the ball in Bakersfield, and he's been searching ever since for.... No, actually, a visionary shoe repairman built this 10-foot-tall shoe in 1947 and installed his shop inside it. The white lace-up oxford measures 32 feet long, has a crisp black sole, and is occupied by the builder's son, who is also a shoe repairman.

BASS LAKE
(45 miles north of Fresno)

Country Summer Games: first Sunday in June, 9 A.M.–4 P.M. Events take place on the village beach, north shore of the lake. For more information, call (209) 642-3676.

Your odds are pretty good at this festival's well-stocked gold-panning troughs. Most oddball event of the day is the "Anything That Floats" contest. We're talking weird boats. A recent competitor paddled a frog-shaped raft while his partner, clad in an aquatic bee costume, swam ahead, pulling the raft on a rope.

BODIE
(30 miles northeast of Lee Vining)

Ghost Town: Go north from Lee Vining 18 miles to Highway 270, the Bodie turnoff. Go up 270 for 13 miles, only the first ten of which are paved. Open Memorial Day–Labor Day, daily, 9 A.M.–7 P.M.; other times open daily, 9 A.M.–4 P.M., but winter conditions can be rough (snow, mud, etc.). Admission: $3 per car. For more information, call (619) 647-6525 or (619) 932-7070.

Bodie is far and away the most impressive abandoned city in California. Now a state historical park, the formerly raucous Bodie looks the way you always imagined a ghost town should look: rickety, leaning wooden buildings; dirt streets and plank sidewalks; rooms full of dust and rotting furniture. Though Bodie is somewhat touristy, and populated by one park ranger, it's not a phony ghost town like Calico or Columbia. All the buildings are authentically unrestored and unmoved, and there's nothing modern in sight except the tourists' cars in the parking lot.

CALIFORNIA CITY
(65 miles east of Bakersfield)

Tortoise Days: first weekend in May. Central Park. For more information, call (619) 373-8676 or (619) 373-4811.

The world's only desert tortoise preserve is in California City. Tortoises live and breed here, officially protected since 1978. Before that, Tortoise Days climaxed with a rip-snorting, though uncool, tortoise race. Nowadays tortoise lovers come to the festival prepared to content themselves with tortoise T-shirts, tortoise-related arts and crafts, tortoise-shaped hats, and exchanges of shaggy-tortoise stories. Recent festival-goers relished the mascot pin, which depicted a you-know-what wearing huarache sandals and a big sombrero.

COALINGA

Decorated Oil Pumps: along Highway 198 north of Coalinga on both sides of the road. Exit Highway 5 west of Coalinga and look for the pumps, starting where Highway 198 joins Highway 33 and turns south. You can't miss the pumps. Always visible. For more information, call the Coalinga Chamber of Commerce at (209) 935-2948.

The animals at the Coalinga Zoo are quite active. Up and down they go. Up and down. And up and down and up and down. This is no ordinary zoo; it's the "Iron Zoo," 60 painted and decorated oil pumps. In 1973 a local artist asked Shell Oil if they'd let her spruce up the then-dreary-looking pumps. They not only let her; they even gave her the paint. The next year, a "create-a-character-for-a-pump" contest expanded the metallic menagerie to include a zebra, grasshopper, bull, cowboy riding a bucking bronco, hobo dog, alligator, eagle that "flies," pink elephant, and 50 more.

Horned Toad Derby: Memorial Day weekend. Races are on Friday evening and all day Saturday and Sunday. Olson Park. For more information, call (209) 935-2948.

Horned toads are not toads but fearsome-looking desert lizards, studded with dinosaurean spikes and nasty claws. Heavy betting precedes each of the races. The toads are placed in the center of a 16-foot circle, and the first toad to scramble to the edge of the circle is the winner. Some toads rocket off the platform in seconds. Occasionally they'll all sit there motionless for endless minutes, like their distant cousins, the iguanas in the zoo. The crowd goes into hysterics trying to get them to move, but no dice.

COLFAX

Bathtub Regatta: usually the last Saturday in July, noon. Greenhorn Park. From Highway 80, take the Colfax turnoff to Highway 174. Greenhorn Park is just off

Highway 174. For more information, call (916) 272-6100.

Anything goes, as long as every craft in the regatta incorporates at least one real bathtub. Recent entrants have included a tub disguised as an airplane and called "Sky Queen, the transvestite son of Sky King". Another, a prissy hot tub, sported balloons and fresh flowers; and the self-explanatory "Hammer and Eggs" was sponsored by a local hardware store and café.

COLUMBIA

Poison Oak Show: fourth Sunday in September, noon. In front of the St. Charles Saloon, corner of Main and Jackson. For more information, call (209) 533-4656.

Yeah, they *know* it's poisonous. That's the whole point. Poison oak grows so exuberantly in this area that the local residents are nicknamed "poison oakers." They feel about the caustic stuff the way the Dutch feel about tulips. Fearless contestants, heavily gloved, fawn over their entries in the following categories: best poison oak arrangement, biggest branch, biggest leaf, most potent-looking green leaves, most potent-looking red leaves, best photo of poison oak, and—no kidding—best bonsai poison oak. Your decision whether or not to attend the festival shouldn't be a rash one.

COULTERVILLE
(30 miles south of Sonora)

Coyote Howling Contest: a weekend in mid-May (varies). Public Park, corner of Main and Stockton Streets. For current date and more information, call (209) 878-3074.

All those nights you've stayed awake howling at the moon were not spent in vain. Compete with people like yourself; throw back your head and make like Wile E. Judging is based, paradoxically, on both originality *and* authenticity. Bring the whole family and compete in the "pack" division. But be warned: Accompanying the Coyote Howl is an event that wins our Illiterate Historical Bogusness award: the incredibly titled Olde Tyme Miner's Country Faire.

FAIRFIELD

The Wright Museum of Space Action: 732 Ohio Street (at Webster Street), central Fairfield. Open by appointment only. Admission: free. Phone: (707) 429-0598.

Any average Joe could tell you Isaac Newton discovered gravity. But he'd be wrong. Newton merely came up with an equation that described gravity. Even to this day nobody has the faintest idea why gravity happens or exactly what it is. Walter Wright is quick to point this out. If gravity is still a total mystery, the Wright Theory of Space Action—to which this museum is dedicated—can't be disproved. Wright's theory is that gravity is a repulsive force rather than an attractive one—a push instead of a pull. Wright has built 75 exhibits and mechanical devices in his house and yard, which, he claims, prove his point of view. Some of these are funny; others are downright confusing.

FIDDLETOWN
(25 miles south of Placerville)

Chinese Herb Shop Museum: downtown Fiddletown, near the corner of Oleta Road and Jibboom Street. Open Saturday, noon–4 P.M. and occasionally by appointment. Admission: free, but donations are welcomed. Phone: (209) 296-4519.

Two herb doctors set up shop in this old adobe in 1850. Their clients were several hundred Chinese gold hunters. The herbs and the doctors are long gone, but the equipment and personal possessions have been carefully preserved. Rows and rows of drawers and cupboards are labeled with the herbs' Chinese names. Also on display are old Chinese calendars, bottles, coins, pipes, and pottery shipped to the Mother Lode from China, via San Francisco.

FRESNO

Storyland: on the western side of Roeding Park, which is bordered by Olive Avenue, North Motel Drive, Belmont Avenue, and Highway 99, in central Fresno. Open May 1–Labor Day, daily, 10 A.M.–5 P.M.; February–April and Labor Day–November, Saturday–Sunday, 10 A.M.–5 P.M. Closed December–January. Admission: $1.75; children under 3, free. Phone: (209) 264-2235.

This verdant fantasyland is greener and more participatory than your average children's park. Don't just look at Jack's beanstalk. Climb it! Get lost in Alice in Wonderland's maze, slide down the Three Bears' slide, and wander the many mysterious paths. The 35 fantasy and folktale vignettes were built, for the most part, in 1960—back when children's park designers knew what they were doing. Don't miss the gigantic miniature (??) King Arthur's Castle, which looks a lot better than the supposedly real King Arthur's Castle in Cadbury, England.

HANFORD

Old Taoist Temple: 12 China Alley (at White Street), second floor. Open by appointment only. Admission: free. Phone: (209) 584-3236 or (209) 584-8860.

Around seven altars you can see old tapestries, teak and marble furniture, plaques, fortune-telling sticks, wood carvings of the Eight Immortals, and other turn-of-the-century Chinese and Chinese-American artifacts. Also in the historic China Alley district are an herb shop and a 100-year-old restaurant.

Renaissance of Kings Faire: first weekend in October; Saturday, 10 A.M.–6 P.M.; Sunday, 10 A.M.–5 P.M. Civic Center Park, 400 North Douty Street (between Fuller and Court). Admission: free. For more information, call (209) 251-9257 or (209) 582-0483.

The clever Hanford faire gets ye olde jump on other California faires. First of all, it doesn't cost anything to get in. Second of all—do you believe this knavery?—it re-creates an earlier historical period. The chosen year is 1520; young King Henry VIII is the jolly sovereign. He's still stuck with his first wife, the hapless Catherine of Aragon, and Elizabeth I is but a glimmer in his eye. Their majesties stroll among the visitors, while diverse characters in Tudor costume dance, sing, jest, and proffer food and crafts.

KINGSBURG
(20 miles southeast of Fresno)

Coffee Pot Water Tower: next to Draper Street in central Kingsburg, adjacent to the city park and the police station; visible from all over the city and from

Highway 99. Always visible. For more information, call (209) 897-2925.

Kingsburg's all-pervasive Swedish theme encompasses every corner of the city. Even the water tower is not immune. Dolled up with an authentically fashioned handle and spout, the huge tank has been painted with traditional Swedish coffee-pot floral designs. "Sven—the water coming out of the kitchen faucet is brown!" "Good. I hope it's decaffeinated this time."

Swedish Festival: third weekend in May. Events take place all over town. For more information, call (209) 897-2925.

About one-third of Kingsburg's residents have Swedish blood coursing through their veins. The town plays this for all it's worth. At the festival you'll find Swedish pancakes, Swedish arts and crafts, children in troll costumes, a lavish Maypole-raising and more. An interesting authentic touch is the traditional pea soup and pancakes dinner, which opens the festival Thursday night.

LEBEC
(37 miles south of Bakersfield)

Civil War Reenactments: third Sunday of every month, April–October. Battles: 10 A.M., noon, and 2 P.M. Parade Ground, Fort Tejon State Historic Park, just north of Lebec. (Take the Fort Tejon turnoff from Highway 5.) Admission: $2; children, 50¢. For more information, call (805) 248-6692.

Civil War buffs around here just couldn't stand having been born 130 years too late, and 2,000 miles too far west. They decided to take action. Now several hundred rebs 'n' yanks descend on the fort once a month to reenact actual Civil War battles. Every detail is correct, from the buttons on the soldiers' uniforms to the blood-curdling instruments in the army doctor's black bag. Also, on the first Sunday of every month, volunteers in Civil War-era costumes "occupy" the historic fort, making the place look just as it did in its heyday.

LEE VINING
(60 miles northwest of Bishop)

Mono Lake Tufa Formations: all along the shores of Mono Lake, east of Lee Vining. The Mono Lake Information Center (east of Lee Vining, next to the lake) gives tours of the formations. The center is open in summer, daily, 9 A.M.–9 P.M.; in winter, daily, 9 A.M.–5 P.M. The formations are always visible. Admission: free. Phone: (619) 647-6595.

The level of Mono Lake used to be higher than it is today. Then the city of Los Angeles, desperate for more water so that its citizens could wash their cars and water their sidewalks every day instead of just four times a week, diverted most of Mono Lake's water sources into the L.A. aqueduct. The lake dropped 46 feet over the next 40 years, exposing the weirdly shaped mineral deposits known as tufa formations. The people who want to save Mono Lake by raising the water level get a lot of publicity and sympathy from all the visitors who come to look at the tufa. But if the lake's level went back up, all the tufa would be underwater. And nobody would visit Mono Lake anymore because its main tourist draw would be underwater. Paradoxical, eh?

LOCKE

(One mile north of Walnut Grove)

Dai Loy Gambling Museum: on River Road, center of town. Open Saturday–Sunday, noon–5 P.M. Admission: voluntary donation. Phone: (916) 775-1048.

Locke is the only town in the United States founded by Chinese people. Lots of tea drinking, gambling, and smoking used to go on in this old building, and the museum is set up to look as if the social hall were still in use and the gamblers had just stepped outside for a breath of air. Fascinating Chinese games, including a keno look-alike complete with numbered ping-pong balls, stand half-played, waiting forever for the gamblers to return.

MODESTO

UFO Exhibit and Library: open by appointment only. Call Marv Taylor at (209) 524-0199 to make appointment and get address. Admission: $2; children 12–18, $1; children under 12, free.

Marv Taylor saw a UFO in 1948, when he was a kid in Oakland, and he's been chasing UFOs ever since. He believes Earth has been visited by aliens, and he has a lot of evidence to support his claim, evidence he's been collecting since 1947—the year UFOs started making regular appearances on Earth. The exhibit (which was in cramped quarters at press time but which will be moving soon) includes 28 display boards showing UFO case histories with photos and text; seven life-size replicas of aliens (based on eyewitness descriptions); tapes of people talking about their experiences with UFOs; over 1,000 rare UFO books; plus articles, videos, and other UFO effluvia.

MURPHYS
(Eight miles northeast of Angels Camp)

Mercer Caverns: 1⅓ miles north of town; follow the signs. (Murphys is just off Highway 4.) Open June–September, daily, 9 A.M.–5 P.M.; October–May, Saturday–Sunday, 11 A.M.–4 P.M. Tours depart every 20 minutes. Admission: $4.50; children, $2.20. Phone: (209) 728-2101.

This staggering vertical cave has been a Mother Lode tourist attraction for more than 100 years. Guided tours go down 440 steps, through ten "rooms," past such suggestive limestone formations as Chocolate Malt, Rapunzel, Polar Bear, Angel Wings, and Chinese Meat Market. The cave is 3 million years old, but in cave terms it's still "alive."

NEVADA CITY

International Teddy Bear Convention: a three-day weekend in late spring (varies). The American Victorian Museum, 325 Spring Street (at Bridge Street). For current dates and other information, call (916) 265-5804.

People don't bring their teddy bears to this convention. The bears bring their people. That's the attitude around here, so fasten your seat-belts: dangerous cuteness ahead. Enthusiastic festival-goers, numbering in the thousands, munch "teddy-bear picnic food," and browse at booths selling teddies and teddy accessories. A prize is awarded to the furthest-traveled bear (*not* to its owner, of course). Meanwhile, Nevada City merchants decorate their shop windows with teddy bears in all sorts of adorable situations. We just hope it isn't terminal.

OAKDALE

Hershey Chocolate Tours: 1400 South Yosemite Avenue (which is Road J14), southern end of town. Open Monday–Friday, 8 A.M.–3 P.M.; closed holidays. Admission: free. Phone: (209) 847-0381.

Switzerland has Lindt, England has Cadbury, Holland has Droste...and all of them look down their noses at American chocolate. Let 'em think what they want. Who's got Hershey's kisses, us or them? Oakdale is the one and only place on earth where you can see Hershey's chocolate being made, so a visit here is, for some, like a pilgrimage to Mecca. See big vats and machines turning out bar after bar, kiss after kiss. And yes, free samples, too.

PLACERVILLE

Toilet Throwing Contest: July 4, in the afternoon (exact time varies). County Fairgrounds, 100 Placerville Drive, on the west side of town; part of the July 4 Blast. For more information, call (916) 626-1222 or (916) 621-5860.

Seasoned toilet throwers compete head to head in a battle for the championship every July 4. Thrown toilets don't go very far; winners and losers are often separated by mere inches. Technique is what counts, not strength. Champions, flushed with their success, walk away with big cash prizes. Is this what they mean by "dry heaves"?

Wagon Train: arrives in Placerville the last weekend in June. Wagon parade down Main Street: Sunday, 11 A.M. For more information, call (916) 621-5885 or (916) 644-6426.

Along the old Emigrant Trail, '49ers found dreams, death, gold, and outrageous bread prices. Now the Emigrant Trail is called Highway 50, and everybody's got ski racks. Would-be '49ers hitch up their own covered wagons every year and spend a week rumbling down the old Emigrant Trail. It's a 30-year tradition. At journey's end, the wagon train rolls into Placerville amid much celebration and hollering. Some families spend all year building their wagons, based on old photos. We doubt, however, that our rugged ancestors' wagons sported—as these do—huge banners with such slogans as "El Dorado Honda."

RANDSBURG

(90 miles east of Bakersfield)

Hard Rock Dinner: in Randsburg Desert Museum, on Butte Avenue, center of town. It's hard to miss. Open Saturday–Sunday and holidays, 10 A.M.–5 P.M. Admission: $1; children, 50¢. No phone.

Most of this museum is the usual local history stuff—mining artifacts and pioneer relics—but one exhibit shines like a beacon of peculiarity: the Hard Rock Dinner. A local bar owner spent years and years out in the desert collecting unusual mineral and geological specimens. After noticing that some of these looked a lot like foodstuffs, he arranged a display in his bar. Now residing in the Randsburg Museum, the Hard Rock Dinner is a complete meal made entirely of rocks: cauliflower, eggs, sausage, pie, potatoes, hamburger—all totally convincing and pretty tasty-looking. They're not carved, but naturally formed rocks, set out on plates and bowls. A comical menu explains the meal. Some like it hard.

RIO VISTA

Foster's Big Horn Saloon: 143 Main Street (at Front). Open Monday, Wednesday, Thursday, and Sunday, 10 A.M.–12:30 A.M.; Tuesday, 10 A.M.–6 P.M.; Friday–Saturday, 10 A.M.–2 A.M. Phone: (707) 374-2511.

Foster's Big Horn has the world's largest one-man collection of animal game trophies. And considering that big-game sport hunting is now illegal just about everywhere, this will always be the world's largest. Former owner Bill Foster bagged 251 unfortunate mammals and brought home his trophies to display in the saloon that supported his safari lifestyle. Foster himself has long since gone to the Happy Hunting Grounds (where angry animal spirits will chase him around till the end of time), but his trophies remain—a veritable zoo of heads.

ROUGH AND READY

(Five miles west of Grass Valley)

Secession Day Celebration: the last Sunday in June. All over town, all day. For more information, call (916) 273-2163.

Rough and Ready is a town with guts. It once was a whole country. In 1850, the U.S. government imposed a tax on all mining claims. Nobody in California was too pleased with the news, especially Rough and Ready. The townspeople got together, unanimously condemned the U.S. government, and seceded from the Union. On April 7 the flag of The Great Republic of Rough and Ready flew over the town. Colonel Brundage was elected president, a constitution was signed, and the folks collectively thumbed their noses at the rest of the country. Rough and Ready lasted only three months as the world's smallest nation. On July 4, swept by a patriotic fervor and maybe feeling a little guilty, they replaced their flag with the Stars and Stripes. Secession Day celebrates the town's brief independence. There's a stage play about the rebellion and wild west mock gunfights.

SACRAMENTO

Best Products Building: 1901 Arden Way, in the Arden Fair Mall, just north of the California Exposition and east of Highway 80. Open Monday–Friday, 9:30 A.M.–9:30 P.M.; Saturday, 10 A.M.–6 P.M.; Sunday, 11 A.M.–6 P.M. Phone: (916) 929-6784.

The Best Products Company hired avant-garde architects to design their stores around the country, and the results were satisfyingly bizarre. When the Sacramento store is closed, it seems to have no front door. But early every morning, a huge, jagged chunk of one of the corners mysteriously slides out a few feet to reveal the hidden entrance. The building, with its removable chunk, looks like it has been struck by an earthquake. Survivors of the disaster take refuge in the damaged structure, entering and exiting through the huge crack in the wall.

Bizarre Collections Exhibit: at the Sacramento History Center, 101 "I" Street (at Front Street) in Old Sacramento. Open only during the month of April (exact dates vary), daily, 10 A.M.–5 P.M. Admission: $2.50; seniors, $1.50; children 6–17, $1; children under 5, free. Phone: (916) 449-2057. To enter the contest, call the Sacramento *Bee* Promotions Department before mid-March at (916) 321-1793.

You may have thought, "I've spent my life obsessively collecting toenail clippings from left-handed bowling champions. Society has no place for me." Not true! Every March, the Sacramento *Bee* and the Sacramento History Center sponsor a contest for the world's most unusual collection. The top three winners are announced in the *Bee*, and all the finalists have their collections exhibited for a month at the History Center. Here's your competition—a few past contest winners: pocket lint, tarantula skins, coffins, potato mashers, copralites, rejection letters from boyfriends, misprinted soda cans, brothel decanters.

Fairytale Town: 3930 W. Land Park Drive, in William Land Park, just south of downtown. Open Monday–Friday, 10 A.M.–5 P.M.; Saturday–Sunday, 10 A.M.–6 P.M. Admission: $1.50; children 3–12, $1; children under 3, free. Phone: (916) 449-5233.

Savvy publicity directors might have named this place "Carl Jung's Dreamland of Subconscious Motifs." Folk tales come to life here in a series of 20 vignettes. The fears, fantasies, and hopes of childhood come back to haunt you as you explore the brightly painted cement-and-fiberglass interpretations of Hansel and Gretel's Gingerbread House, the Crooked Man and his Crooked Mile, Old Mother Hubbard, Cinderella, and a generic central European-style castle to fill in for all the folk tales they missed.

Fiberglass Menagerie: 7539 Power Inn Road, south of Florin Road, southeast end of town, in the equipment yard owned by Duke Cahill. Always somewhat visible from the street, but the yard itself is never open to visitors.

Take some discarded fiberglass. Add a few hundred gallons of plaster and a truckload of plastic barrels. Mix well with a pinch of inspiration and know-how. What have you got? A yard bursting with towering fantasy animals in bewildering shapes. One mythical wild creature stands 30 feet tall and has eyes that glow at night.

Thermometer Museum: 4555 Auburn Boulevard, Suite 11 (at Pasadena, in the northern part of the city). Open Monday–Friday, 9 A.M.–6 P.M. Admission: free. Phone: (916) 487-6964.

You've probably been wondering what happens to all of the world's egg incubation thermometers when they've been put out to pasture. Look no further. They're here, in the world's largest collection of thermometers: thermometers mounted in ivory, gold, brass, and even stranger media; thermometers shaped like cupids, bi-cycles, churches; thermometers designed by Tiffany. The collection spans 200 years and half the globe.

SAN ANDREAS

Underground Lake Trips: California Caverns, nine miles east of town. Take Mountain Ranch Road from San Andreas, and follow the signs. Tours by reservation only, mid-May–November. Admission: $49. Phone: (209) 736-2708.

John Muir marveled at this underground lake a century ago and was moved to write that "its eternal calm excites the imagination even more profoundly than the silvery lakes of the glaciers." The five-hour tour, called the Downstream Circuit, lets you raft across the subterranean lake. Then you get to crawl on your belly through muddy passages, as only your illuminated hat stands between you and total darkness. (Other tours, both more and less extravagant, are also available. The more extravagant ones, however, require previous caving experience.)

SELMA

Raisin Festival: first Saturday in May, 10:30 A.M.–6 P.M. Most events take place at Pioneer Village, northwest of town, off Highway 99. For more information, call (209) 896-3315.

We were hoping to find a raisin look-alike contest at this festival, but we found a forklift rodeo. Drivers maneuver their way through an obstacle course—first forward, then backward. The competitors also demonstrate their stacking and loading techniques. Wahoo! Also on the agenda are a raisin tray-turning contest and a raisin recipe contest. Be warned: Selma is the Raisin Capital of the world. Folks around here have been known to slip raisins into brownies, turkey salad, three-bean salad, relish, and even—gasp—spaghetti sauce.

SEQUOIA NATIONAL PARK

Wacky Logs: From Visalia, drive east on Highway 198 through Three Rivers, where it becomes Generals Highway; when you get to Giant Forest Village, turn right (south) on Crescent Meadow Road. All three logs are along this road (see below). Always open. Admission: free. Phone: (209) 561-3314.

The trees in Sequoia National Park are the largest living things in the world. And when they fall down and die, they're the largest dead things in the world. Naturally, man has wrought his will on a few of these gargantuan logs.

The Auto Log: Nine-tenths of a mile south of Giant Forest Village on the north side of the road is a short spur road that leads to the so-called Auto Log. No, it's not shaped like a car; it's flattened on top so you can drive your auto onto it. This is well known as the primary funny-photo spot in the park.

The Tunnel Log: 1½ miles further along the Crescent Meadow Road is the Tunnel Log. Don't worry about missing it—the log is lying right across the road. A tunnel was carved sideways through it in 1938 to allow access to the rest of the park. In northern California, people drive through upright living trees. Here in the south they're content to drive through prone logs.

Tharp's Log: Drive to the end of Crescent Meadow Road and park. Walk along the south Crescent Meadow Trail for one mile; the trail goes right past the log. Hale Tharp, the first white man ever to see these giant sequoias, built his house inside a huge hollow fallen log. The main room is 56 feet long and eight feet high. It's still there, even after 130 years. Gives a new meaning to the words "tree house."

SODA SPRINGS

Western America Skisport Museum: at Boreal Ski Area, ten miles west of Truckee, off Highway 80. Open in summer, Wednesday–Sunday 11 A.M.–5 P.M.; in winter, Tuesday–Sunday, 11 A.M.–5 P.M. Admission: free. Phone: (916) 426-3313.

Faced with lots of snow, Scandinavian prospectors made themselves cross-country skis back in the 1850s, patterned after the ones they had worn at home. People have been skiing in the Sierras ever since. The museum displays miners' skis, horses' snowshoes, and vintage ski "dopes" (waxes) and their once-secret recipes. You'll also learn about the WWII "ski troopers" who fought in Italy, and about "Snowshoe" Thompson, gold-rush-era skiing postman and one-man Pony Express.

STOCKTON

Pixie Woods: in Louis Park, near the end of Monte Diablo Avenue, next to the ship channel at the west side of town, on Pixie Drive. Open March–May, Saturday–Sunday, noon–5 P.M.; June–September, Wednesday–Friday, 11 A.M.–5 P.M.; Saturday–Sunday, 11 A.M.–6 P.M.; September–October, Saturday–Sunday, noon–5 P.M.; closed November–February. Admission: $1; children under 12, 75¢; rides, 50¢. Phone: (209) 944-8220.

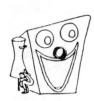

It's at places like this that kids learn about life and the real world. "That's Neptune, darling, God of the Sea. Nobody believes in him anymore." "The pirate is dressed that way because he is gay. You'll learn about that later, in sex education class." "Yes, people used to ride paddlewheeled boats in the Delta, but there weren't any volcanoes like this one." Plenty of surrealistic mini-buildings further distort the young ones' vision of reality—such as a ten-foot-high, lopsided, blue, grinning telephone.

Wonderful World of Windmills: 6553 Waterloo Road (which is Highway 88), about two miles northeast of town. (Look for palm trees and windmills.) Always visible. Admission: free, but the owner charges "$10 or $20 if you wanna take a picture."

From the road you can see what might be the world's largest windmill collection. Should you brave the "No Trespassing" signs and chained, barking dogs, and go into the yard to talk windmills with the owner, be prepared for a ride into conversational never-never land. "My wife left me after 47 years," he half brags, half laments. "I'm 82 and I got all my teeth and no cavities. That's a world's record." "Been on TV 23 or 24 times." "Spent $9,000 on that 20-foot mill." If you're patient, he'll tell you as much about windmills as you ever wanted to know and more. Recommendation: Stay behind the fence and ogle from there.

TAFT
(30 miles west of Bakersfield)

West Kern Oil Museum: south of downtown on Wood Street, where it intersects with Highways 119 and 113. (Look for the tall wooden oil derrick.) Open Tuesday,

9:30 A.M.–4 P.M.; Wednesday and Saturday–Sunday, 1–4 P.M.; Friday, 9:30 A.M.–noon. Admission: free. Phone: (805) 765-6664.

Oil drilling is fascinating in its own right. Right? But where else but the West Kern Oil Museum can you find a "talking" exhibit on the Great Taft Mouse Invasion of 1924? Thousands of crazed rodents reared up out of the nearby fields and attacked the town as residents feverishly dug moats in an attempt to drown them. The Taft air echoed with startled cries, squeaks, the whirr of lashing tails...and suddenly the mice turned around and went home, just as abruptly as they had come. Hey, don't miss the tar pit exhibit.

THREE RIVERS
(25 miles east of Visalia)

Rock Canyon Llama Ranch: Three Rivers is a resort town on Highway 198, at the entrance to Sequoia National Park. Call beforehand and the rancher, Mrs. Johnson, will meet you in town and take you to the ranch. Admission: free. Phone: (209) 561-4245 (evenings) or (209) 561-4535 (days).

The one-hour tour lets you get really close to llamas: You can feed them, lead them around, pet the babies, and learn about why people are taking them on pack trips into the mountains. Along with the 15 or so llamas, you can also meet and feed black Australian swans.

TRUCKEE

Donner Party Museum: in Donner Memorial State Park, 12593 Donner Pass Road, two miles west of Truckee. From Highway 80, take the Donner State Park exit. Open in summer, daily, 10 A.M.–4 P.M.; in winter, daily, 10 A.M.–noon and 1–4 P.M. Admission: $1; children 6–17, 50¢; children under 6, free. Phone: (916) 587-3841.

If the Donner party had come along a hundred years later, they'd be a cult movie. This museum houses personal relics of the ill-fated wagon train, which was snowbound in the Sierras and forced by hunger into cannibalism. On display are party members' clothes, letters, and parts of their wagons. For real aficionados, there's the chisel on which George Donner cut his hand, thus setting into motion his own gangrenous death. What's for dessert?

Snow Sculpture and Ice Carving: at Snowfest, ten days in early March (varies). Activities take place all around the north shore of Lake Tahoe. Snow palace is at Boreal Ski Area. Ice carving is in Tahoe City, first Saturday of the festival, 9 A.M.–noon. For current dates and more information, call (916) 583-7625.

Every year a palace rises from the gleaming snow. A Scottish castle, a Norman fortress...the design is different each year. Built by experts and made of pure snow, the palaces measure about 40 by 70 feet. Meanwhile, chefs compete in the ice-carving spectacular, creating chilly masterworks. Other festival events include the crowning of a lovely Mr. Lake Tahoe, a dress-up-your-dog contest, and—brrr!—dancing in the street.

TULARE

Bed Race: on a Saturday in mid-July. On Tulare Avenue, center of town. Race starts at 9 A.M. For current date call (209) 688-2011.

Bed racing in Tulare is a serious matter. Beds are customized at high-performance auto repair shops; special racing wheels are welded on; racers build up their muscles for weeks beforehand. All for a 100-yard race. Judging is based not only on speed but also on engineering. Who says bed races are for wimps?

Reptile World, USA: 110 North Mooney Boulevard (at Tulare Boulevard). Open daily, 10 A.M.–6 P.M. Admission: $5.75; students and seniors, $5.25; children, $4.75; children under 2, free. Phone: (209) 688-0561.

With more than 3,000 scaly scamps on hand, this might be the world's largest reptile collection. At any rate you'll see enough beady eyes, darting tongues, and detachable tails to make you glad you're a large mammal. Snakes, alligators, and lizards make for tons of cold-blooded fun. Give a cheery hello to Snidely, the four-foot-long iguana.

TURLOCK

Bulldozer Building: the United Equipment Company, 600 West Glenwood Avenue, next to Lander Avenue and Highway 99, southern edge of town. Always visible. Phone: (209) 632-9931.

Extensive research convinces us that this is the only bulldozer-shaped building in the whole wide—and soon to be flat—world. And it's not just life-size, either. It's about ten times life-size, and it houses the office complex of a company that sells bulldozers and caterpillars. The building's extensive and realistic details include handgrip shifting gears, hydraulic lifts, exhaust pipes, treads, and a seat.

VACAVILLE

Onion Festival: a weekend in early to mid-September (varies). In the Pena Adobe Park, southwest of town, just south of Highway 80. Events are on Saturday from 10 A.M.–7 P.M., Sunday 10 A.M.–6 P.M. Admission to festival grounds: $4; children 3–12 and seniors, $2; children under 3, free. Phone (707) 448-6424.

Other cities might be a little more closed-mouthed about being a major onion-processing center—if only to duck a predictable barrage of bad-breath jokes. But Vacaville is proud. "Onion juices course through our veins," brags a Vacaville brochure. "The city smells like a giant caldron of onion soup!" This frenzy of onion pride climaxes with the festival's cooking "dem-onion-stra-tions" and a Wheel of "Fortu-onion." Don't miss the tear-jerking raw-onion-eating championship, with prelimi-naries on Saturday and finals on Sunday.

The Wooz: 500 Orange Drive, just south of Highway 80 at Lawrence Drive, near the Nut Tree, northeast of town. Open daily, 10 A.M.–10 P.M. Admission: $7; children 5–12, $4.50; children under 5, free; seniors over 55, $5. Phone: (707) 446-5588.

American maze-lovers have long lamented the sorry state of the U.S. maze scene. Britain has dozens of human-sized hedge mazes; we have almost none. Along comes the Wooz to remedy the situation. This is America, so the Wooz is made of redwood, not hedges, and reaps a nifty profit besides. The Wooz (which, in-comprehensibly, stands for Wild Original Object of Zoom) is actually three mazes: the simple Mini-Wooz; The Wooz; and the Super Wooz, a gigantic maze for geniuses and hyperactive children. People who finish in the best times are invited back to compete in the maze championships. The best part is that they change the mazes constantly by moving the redwood panels, so every time you come back you're facing a new Wooz.

VALLECITO
(Four miles northeast of Angels Camp)

Moaning Cavern: 5350 Moaning Cave Road, just off Parrotts Ferry Road and Highway 4; eight miles north of Columbia State Park; five miles east of Angels Camp. Open in summer, daily, 9 A.M.–6 P.M.; in winter, daily, 10 A.M.–5 P.M. Admission: $5; children 6–12, $2.50; children under 6, free. Phone: (209) 736-2708.

A 100-foot steel stairway spirals into the cave's depths, and eerie moans swirl about your head. Prosaically, the moans are not the cries of the long-dead humans whose bones were discovered here in 1851, but an effect of water dripping in holes in the cave's walls. The old bones are still on view here, as are such formations as the 30-foot "Igloo" and 14-foot "Pendulum." Don't like spiral staircases? For $19 you can rappel down the side—180 feet—with a rope. No experience necessary. If you make it, they give you a "survivor" card. On the three-hour Adventure Tour ($35, by reservation only) you rappel as well as explore hidden, undeveloped parts of the cavern.

VISALIA

Restaurant Race: third Thursday in July; course is on Main Street between Locust Avenue and West Street. Races start at 7:30 P.M. Phone: (209) 732-7737.

Visalia has taken to waiters' and waitresses' races in a big way. Though their first race was as recent as 1985, they're already attracting runners from as far away as Fresno, they've established a fast-food division, they enforce strict dress codes, and they have special judges who keep a keen eye out for cheaters. The waiters and waitresses must balance two full wine glasses and a bottle on a tray (no spilling allowed) as they scramble up and back the three-block course. Fast-food workers balance a cup of soda pop and a hamburger.

THE SAN FRANCISCO BAY AREA

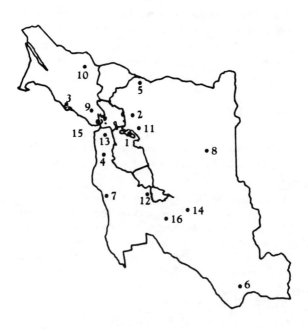

Legend:

1. Alameda
2. Berkeley
3. Bolinas
4. Colma
5. Crocket
6. Gilroy
9. Mill Valley
10. Novato
11. Oakland
12. Palo Alto
13. San Franciscot
14. San Jose

The mere word "city" is inadequate to describe San Francisco. It shimmers in our minds, a mythical place of romance and fantasy, as perfectly unreal as Shangri-La or Atlantis. Even long-time residents, who know full well that San Francisco is not immune to the problems that plague all large cities, still can't help but think of their hometown as magically, beautifully unreal, regardless of the fact that their Toyota just got flattened by a cable car and their wife ran off with a moody poet.

Cities cluster around the bay, seemingly jostling for position to bask in San Francisco's beneficent glow. But this isn't like other places where the entire metropolitan area is dismissively dubbed "Los Angeles" or "London" or "New York", thereby denying the individuality of the neighboring cities. In the Bay Area, each city has a strong identity and a unique personality. If you grew up in Yonkers or Santa Monica you'd say that you were from New York or Los Angeles; if you grew up in Sausalito or Berkeley it would be unthinkable to say that you were from San Francisco. Whether this is due to pride in one's own hometown or respect for the well-defined image of San Francisco depends on your point of view.

ALAMEDA

Sand Castle Contest: a Saturday in early June (date varies), 9 A.M.–1 P.M. At Robert Crown Memorial Beach, Otis Drive at Westline Drive. For exact date and more information, call (415) 531-9300, ext. 2208.

There's no crashing surf at this beach; so for 20 years, would-be architects have created their own scenery. Adults, children, and entire families compete. Recent entries have included a languorous mermaid, some wallowing hippos, a chubby tugboat, a dragon-haunted castle, and the "Sandy 500" race car.

ALCATRAZ
(One mile north of San Francisco)

Alcatraz Prison Tours: Ferries leave from San Francisco's Pier 41 (next to Jefferson Street and Powell Street) in summer, daily, from 8:15 A.M. to 4:15 P.M., every half hour at 15 and 45 minutes after the hour; in winter, daily, from 8:45 A.M. to 2:45 P.M. every hour at 45 minutes after the hour. Price: with cassette tape commentary, $7; seniors, $6.50; children, $4.50; without cassette tape commentary, $5; seniors, $4.50; children, $3. Phone: (415) 546-2896.

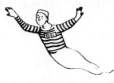

The inmates are long gone. Even the ghosts of the inmates have been chased away by the steady stream of curious sightseers. Yet Alcatraz still has a certain macabre charm, a siren's song of murder and mystery that is plenty hard to resist. The cassette tape guided tour fills you in on the history and legends, but the headphones and droning voices interfere with the point of an Alcatraz visit: to drink in the desolate atmosphere of the place. You can stay on the crumbling, windblown island as long as you like, but be forewarned that the last boat back leaves at 6:05 P.M. in summer and 4:35 P.M. in winter.

ANGEL ISLAND
(One mile southeast of Tiburon)

Abandoned Garrisons: Ferries leave from San Francisco's Pier 41 (next to Jefferson Street and Powell Street) Monday–Friday, 10 A.M. (return ferry at 2:50 P.M.); Saturday, Sunday, and holidays, 10 A.M., 2 P.M. and 3:45 P.M. (last return ferry at 4:25 P.M.). Price: $7.10; children, $4.05. Phone: for the ferries: (415) 546-2896; for the Angel Island Ranger Station: (415) 435-1915.

Angel Island is the Bay Area's island-of-all-trades. It has, over the years, been a Civil War military fort, a troop embarcation point, an immigrant quarantine station, a Nike missile base, an Indian village, a hideout for a brothel, and a state park. Many remnants of the island's previous lives still remain. You can explore the abandoned military buildings at Camp Reynolds, and scour other buildings for graffiti left by anxious soldiers and Asian immigrants. Inquire at the ranger station near the debarcation point (Ayala Cove) for directions to the various ruins.

BERKELEY

Bible Collection: in the Badé Institute of Biblical Archaeology, a brick and masonry building on the east side of the Pacific School of Religion campus, 1798 Scenic Avenue (at Le Conte Avenue, just a few blocks north of the University of California campus). Open Monday–Friday, 9 A.M.–noon and 1–4:30 P.M. Admission: free. Phone (415) 848-0528.

Some of the treasures in this unusual collection include a first-edition 1611 King James Bible, a 1535 Coverdale Bible (the first to be printed in English), and a 1536 Tyndale New Testament. The collection, assembled over a lifetime by a local rare books dealer, includes nearly 300 gorgeously printed Bibles in many languages.

Krishna Parade: on a Sunday in late March or early April (date varies); starts at noon at Bancroft Way and Telegraph Avenue, and continues down Telegraph to Willard Park at Derby Street and Regent Street. For exact date and more information, call (415) 540-9215.

This extravagant procession honors Lord Chaitanya, founder of the Krishna movement. A 20-foot-high statue of Chaitanya is wheeled reverently down the street as revelers hand out free food and heavy doses of Krishna consciousness.

May Day Morris Dancing: May 1, at dawn. At Inspiration Point, off Wildcat Canyon Road at the eastern edge of Tilden Regional Park.

Morris is a clomping, bell-jingling style of dance, usually associated with little British villages. But that doesn't stop Berkeley from having its very own Morris troupe. In the eerie half dark, everyone's welcome to watch them "dance up the dawn." The dancers, clad in crisp red and white, thump and stomp their way through the old May Day fertility dances. What you do in the woods before and afterward is entirely your own business.

Wind Pipes: at the top of Centennial Drive, on the eastern edge of the University of California campus; from Gayley Road, turn east onto Stadium Rimway and then left on Centennial. Wind pipes are just behind the Lawrence Hall of Science, on the hillside facing the bay (west). Visible anytime. For more information, call (415) 642-5132.

Thirty-one metal pipes loom spookily up and out of the earth like baleful armless saguaros. Slits cut into the cylinders create mournful music when the wind blows through: subtle; melancholy with a touch of church bells; thoroughly appropriate to this often cold, foggy hillside.

The pipes command a sweeping bay view—with mood music, gratis.

BUTTERFLY TREES

This is where migrating Monarch butterflies spend their winters in the Bay Area.

Bolinas: on Terrace Avenue, next to Bolinas Bay, in the eucalyptus trees that hang over the street. Phone: (415) 388-2595.

Prime butterfly season here is from October to February.

Muir Beach: From Bolinas, go south ten miles on Highway 1. Park at the Muir Beach parking lot and walk about one block east until you come to a set of stairs; climb the stairs and look for a Monterey pine grove. Phone: (415) 388-2595.

This insect resort area actually has a name: The Elizabeth Terwilliger Butterfly Grove. As noted above, October to February is the time to visit.

COLMA

(Two miles south of San Francisco)

Pet's Rest Cemetery: 1905 Hillside Boulevard. Open Monday–Friday, 9 A.M.–5 P.M.; Saturday, 10 A.M.–2 P.M. Phone: (415) 755-2201.

Colma draws its share of ghoulish mirth hereabouts. It's the graveyard town—nearly all its acreage is given over to cemeteries and nearly all of its residents are dead. This is where San Franciscans go when, instead of passing over the Golden Gate, they pass through the Pearly Gates. Colma has an Italian cemetery, a Chinese cemetery, a Catholic cemetery, and, among others, a pet cemetery. Wander around these dozen bittersweet acres and contemplate 48 years of pet death.

CROCKETT

Neon: Victorian Antiques: 1400 Pomona Street. Open daily, 11 A.M.–5 P.M. Phone: (415) 787-2372. *Another Time Antiques:* 1326 Pomona Street. Open daily, 11 A.M.–5 P.M. Phone: (415) 787-2960. *Tubes of Mystery:* 628 2nd Avenue (upstairs) at Ceres, north of Pomona

Street. Open daily, 10 A.M.–8 P.M. Phone: (415) 787-2446.

Tiny Crockett boasts more neon than certain West African nations. Most of the glow is on Pomona Street, where antique stores specialize in vintage neon signs. Another Time Antiques, from whom Lucasfilm has rented neon signs to use in its movies, has a modest collection of truly unusual specimens, including one depicting a svelte lady diving into a pool. Victorian Antiques fairly bursts with figural neon signs—over 200 of them, including stars, bottles, ice-cream cones, and pizza slices. The owner's prized possession is a 40-square-foot orange cow with a pink cowbell. Tubes of Mystery, meanwhile, is a local neon artist's 600-square-foot brainchild. It goes through a complicated sequence of winks and patterns, and glows the weirdest colors you've ever seen.

EMERYVILLE
(Between Oakland and Berkeley, on the bay)

Emeryville Mudflats: just west of Highway 880, south of Powell Street and north of the Bay Bridge on-ramp; visible from the freeway. To get there on foot, park near the vicinity of Powell Street and the frontage road on the west side of the highway; walk south along the frontage road (and wear boots). Always visible. Admission: free.

The best known and—in a certain sense—most unique of the Bay Area's public artworks are the sculptures on the Emeryville mudflats. Well-known is an understatement: They stand alongside the most heavily trafficked freeway this side of L.A. Folk sculptures like this are usually the product of one person, laboring to satisfy his or her own personal muse; not so in Emeryville. Anybody willing to brave the mud can tromp out there and create something out of driftwood that a million people will see every day. And for every new sculpture that goes up, the wind and tides topple an old one. It's an ever-changing sculpture garden with no rules.

GILROY

Garlic Festival: last weekend in July; gates open at 10 A.M. on all three days. At Christmas Hill park, southwest edge of town. Signs from Highway 101 direct you to the festival and to sites where you can catch a free shuttle bus to the festival. Admission: on Friday, $5; children and seniors, $1; Saturday and Sunday, $6 each day; children and seniors, $2. For more information, call (408) 842-1625.

Garlic—everybody's favorite aphrodisiac, cold remedy, and vermifuge—gets more than its share of attention at this famous festival, which got its start in 1979 when some locals heard of a popular garlic fête at a village in France. "Hey," growled the Gilroy bunch, "we've got a lot more garlic then *they* have!" At Gilroy's festival, you can sample all kinds of garlic-rich food. Watch—and sniff—the Great Garlic Cook-off; buy a real garlic necklace, headband, belt buckle, or other token to show your allegiance to what folks around here call "the stinking rose."

The Tree Circus: in the Enchanted Forest in Hecker Pass amusement park, 3050 Hecker Pass Highway (Highway 152). From Highway 101 in Gilroy take the Leavesley Road exit, and, following the signs for Highway 152, turn left on Monterey for one block and then right on Hecker Pass Highway. Continue west for three miles until you come to Uvas Creek; there will be construction and an entrance to what looks like a plant nursery (unless you're reading this after spring 1990, when the park will—supposedly—be open). Drive in and say you want to see the Tree Circus. Open daily, 9 A.M.–5 P.M.; making an appointment may help. Admission: free (unless, of course, you're reading this after spring 1990). Phone: (408) 842-2121.

Axel Erlandson, a self-taught horticulturalist and un-

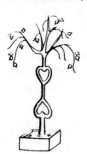

recognized genius, discovered in 1925 a technique with which he could make trees grow into any shape he desired. For the next 40 years he grew 70 trees so incredible in form and design that no words do them justice: living chairs, ladders, double curlicues, spirals, cages, and loops within loops. Long a tourist attraction north of Santa Cruz, the amazing trees stood forgotten after Erlandson died. Many of the trees also died— of neglect. Twenty-eight surviving trees were recently bought and moved to Gilroy, where they will become an attraction at Hecker Pass amusement park. As of this writing, the park isn't open yet, but the unofficial word is that drop-in visitors—if they ask nicely—will be shown the trees. In a word, they're mind-boggling: Go see for yourself.

HALF MOON BAY
(20 miles south of San Francisco, on the coast)

Architectural Potpourri: at the Miramar Beach Health Center, at 1 Mirada Road, in Miramar. From Half Moon Bay go north 2½ miles on Highway 1 until you come to Miramar; turn left (west) on Medio Avenue toward the ocean. From Medio Avenue turn left on Mirada Road and continue until it ends. Always visible.

A cement angel stands on the peak of an A-frame house, wings carrying her back to heaven, where she'll report on things terrestrial: "Sir, they're making some very strange buildings down there." The enclave of peculiarity she's leaving behind includes a massage studio in a landlocked Norwegian fishing boat with stairs cut into the side, a geodesic dome, tipis, bizarre carvings, a boulder suspended from a gate's crosspiece, and a lot of unconventional people.

House of Doors: three miles inland from Half Moon Bay on Highway 92; the house is at an extremely sharp turn, on the north side of the road, across the road from the Obester Winery. Always visible.

At first it doesn't look like much. If you can find a place to park (not an easy task), walk up for a closer look. This entire ramshackle house is constructed of nothing but doors. Only a few actually *open:* the rest are used as walls. Built by a woman named Anne Howe (thus usually referred to as Anne Howe's House of Doors), its unusual design is supposedly nothing more than an accident of fate. Ms. Howe acquired some doors left over from the Pan American Exposition in 1915, wanted to build a house but had no building materials, and...you can guess the rest.

Pumpkin Festival: third weekend in October, 10 A.M.– 5 P.M. both days. Great Pumpkin Parade is at noon on Saturday down Miramontes Street. Pumpkin Pie-Eating Contest is on Saturday, 2:30 and 4 P.M., and Sunday, 3 P.M., at the IDES Grounds on Main Street. Pumpkin Carving Contest is on Sunday, 10 A.M.–1 P.M., at the IDES Grounds. For more information, call (415) 726-5202 or (415) 726-3491.

Okay, so you won't be alone here. Three hundred thousand visitors make the pilgrimage to this event every year—desperate, we suppose, to get a glimpse of the year's largest pumpkin, selected the previous week at a ceremonious "weigh-in." (A recent winner weighed over 600 pounds.) Everything's an orange blur at the Pumpkin Pie-Eating Contest, and everybody's making funny faces at the Pumpkin Carving Contest—all in honor of our chubby, seed-filled pal.

LIVERMORE

World's Longest-Lasting Light Bulb: in Fire Station #1, 4550 East Avenue, at Almond Avenue, on the east side of town. In the fire truck garage area. Always visible. Admission: free. Phone: (415) 373-5461.

These are the days of planned obsolescence. Light bulbs are purposely designed to burn out after a year or two—so the company can sell more replacement bulbs. Ninety years ago companies didn't have modern business sense: They naïvely built the best product they could. In 1901 Shelby Electric Co. made a hand-blown bulb with a carbide filament. It was installed in a Livermore fire station, where it still burns to this day. The yellowish light from its convoluted filament competes feebly with nearby banks of fluorescent bulbs. This bulb is *proof* that they don't make 'em like they used to.

LOS ALTOS HILLS
(Five miles west of Sunnyvale)

Electronics Museum: Foothill College, where Highway 280 and El Monte Road intersect; from Highway 280 take the El Monte Road exit. Museum is next to the observatory, northwest corner of the campus, on College Loop Road. Open Thursday–Friday, 9:30 A.M.–4:30 P.M.; Sunday, 1–4 P.M. Admission: free. Phone: (415) 960-4383.

After ten years of dormancy, this educational museum is being lovingly restored. Science buffs of all ages will get a jolt out of the many hands-on exhibits that explore electricity and magnetism. Especially shocking is the Tesla Coil, which makes an eight-inch spark and lights up the room. A 16th-century electrostatic machine makes plenty of sparks, too. Habitués of electronics-happy Silicon Valley might want to spend their coffee breaks here.

MILL VALLEY

The Unknown Museum: 243 East Blithedale Avenue, near Dell Street, on the north side of the street; from Highway 101, get off at the East Blithedale exit and head west for 1½ miles. Open Sunday, noon–6 P.M. Admission: free. Phone: (415) 383-2726. The museum may have moved by the time you read this; to find its new location call the above number or (415) 388-9700.

The Unknown Museum, in a quest for America's soul, has instead stumbled on its funnybone. The artifacts of 40 years of American culture fill every room, every closet, and even the yard of an overgrown two-story house. The exhibits—perhaps "explosions" would be a better word—are grouped thematically, according to what room they're in. Thus, the kitchen has mountains of plastic fruit, white bread nailed to the wall, and appliances of dubious function; the boy's room contains stacks of old board games and shelf after shelf of war toys; the bathroom is a display of toothbrushes and toilet paper. And everywhere you look are TVs, plastic dolls, and more TVs. Visitors, awash in a sea of childhood memories, often leave thinking about their own lives instead of the museum.

NOVATO

The Renaissance Pleasure Faire: for six weekends in fall, usually from late August or early September to early October, Saturday, Sunday, and Labor Day, 10 A.M.–6 P.M. From Highway 101, turn north on Highway 37 between Ignacio and Novato; after two miles get off at the Atherton/Black Point exit and turn right on Renaissance Road; you'll see the faire from the highway, so it's hard to get lost. Admission: $11.50; students and seniors, $8.50; children under 12, $4.50. Phone: (415) 781-4646 or (415) 892-0937.

The 16th century comes to life for six merry weeks each year in a Marin County forest turned Renaissance village. Thousands of actors, craftspeople and plain common folk polish up their Queen's English and spend days thinking, acting, speaking, and living in Elizabethan England. Of all the Renaissance faires across the land, this one gets our nod as the most heavily researched, largest, and most overwhelming. On our last visit we noticed a few peculiar discrepancies creeping in (such as Japanese food, midway games, and fur-clad Teutonic barbarians straight out of the Dark Ages), though for the most part the ambience is authentic down to the last detail.

OAKLAND

Bathtub Regatta: a Saturday usually in early August (exact date depends on the tides), noon–5 P.M. At San Leandro Regional Shoreline Park: the east-facing beach, off Doolittle Drive, across the water from the Oakland Coliseum. For current date and more information, call (415) 652-9202.

Three dozen well-dressed tubs struggle and splash along a 200-yard saltwater race course. Prizes are awarded to the Fastest High-Tech Tub, Funniest Tub, and Most Creative Tub. Recent entries included a Viking-ship tub; a Harley-Davidson tub; and Wacky Ducky, a duck-headed bathtub complete with yellow feathers and black bow tie.

The Bone Room: at press time, the Bone Room was in transit, searching for new quarters and operating on an appointment-only basis. For new address and/or to make an appointment, call (415) 465-5400.

The next time you need two dozen rat skulls to hand out as party favors, give the Bone Room a call. Want something bigger—a rabbit skull, a mink skull, a horse skull? Something exotic—a wildebeest skull, a warthog skull? Something, oh, I don't know, indulgent—a Cape buffalo skull at $350? These folks sell diverse animal bones as well as bone jewelry, bone books, and insects. It's Grandma's birthday, didja say?

The Bulwinkle House: 5333 Manila Avenue, just west of College Avenue, near Clifton Street. Always visible.

The Bulwinkle House is most definitely a strange edifice, the kind of unexpected vision of quirkiness that we appreciate. The whole place is bristling with metal cutout sculptures, many of them perched high on poles. Disturbing, rusty faces peer from every angle. Bicycle wheels spin in the breeze. Animals, vehicles, boats, bones, bodies, flowers, and unidentifiable shapes form a metal forest that almost totally obscures the house. A glowering sun surveys the tangle from atop the tallest pole. Mr. Bulwinkle is considering taking down his work, so go see it before it disappears. (Remember, this is a private residence; don't disturb the occupants or the art under any circumstances.)

Children's Fairyland: in Lakeside Park, on the north side of Lake Merritt, near Grand Avenue and Parkview. Open daily, 10 A.M.–5:30 P.M. (gates close at 5 P.M.). Admission: $2; children 1–12, $1.50; children under 1, free. Phone: (415) 832-3609.

A sign at the entrance to Children's Fairyland states that adults are not allowed into the park *unless accompanied by a child*. A joke, right? Think again. The rule is strictly enforced. Fairyland was designed solely with tots in mind, and 1950s tots at that, so the adult rules of normality just don't apply. Boldly painted plaster statues act out disturbingly familiar scenes from folktales and nursery rhymes. Weird, tiny, dysfunctional buildings cover the landscape. And a bulbous teapot-castle is home to California's most unusual post office, just wide enough for an adult to turn around in. It sports its own "Children's Fairyland" postmark.

Della's China Cup Café: 7309 MacArthur Boulevard, at 73rd Avenue. Open Monday–Friday, 7 A.M.–3 P.M.; Saturday 7 A.M.–2 P.M. Phone: (415) 569-8112.

You'd think the world's largest teacup collection would be in the Smithsonian Institute or somewhere in England. Would you believe across the street from the Eastmont Mall? The walls of Della's China Cup Café are lined with over 2,000 teacups. The owner, Della herself, has traveled far and wide, tracking down cups for her enormous collection. Devoted friends and patrons have contributed cups, and now Della has about 3,000 in all, though she only has enough room to display 2,000. How many other East Bay eateries have been mentioned in *Ripley's Believe It or Not?*

Gingerbread House Restaurant: 741 5th Street (at Castro Street), just northwest of Jack London Square. Open for lunch and dinner Tuesday–Saturday, by reservation only. Price range: $15.95–$34.95. Phone: (415) 444-7373.

The woman who runs this place heard a folktale about a gingerbread man when she was a tot in Louisiana. Now her fantasy-come-true restaurant (in a complex called

Gingerland) fairly explodes with gingerbread imagery. Hand-painted gingerbread men dance all over the walls, inside and out, playing the saxophone, shimmying with crayfish, wearing chefs' hats, and stirring pots of jambalaya. Hundreds of gingerbread-man dolls in international costumes decorate the restaurant. In a shop downstairs you can buy gingerbread-scented soap and bubble bath. Everywhere are cunningly painted, dizzying constellations of cookies, candies, red hearts, moons, bluebirds—and the urgent reminder: "We Love You."

Harbor Tours: May–August, Thursdays only. Times vary. Meet the boat in Jack London Square, between Scott's Seafood (73 Jack London Square) and The Grotto (70 Jack London Square). Admission: free. Phone: (415) 839-7488.

Maybe nobody's ever written any songs about it, but Oakland's harbor is bigger and busier than San Francisco's. During the 90-minute tour, you glide around in a boat as the tour guide explains how harbors work, what ships do, and what kinds of products travel back and forth across the seas.

OLEMA
(11 miles northwest of Bolinas)

Earthquake Trail: starts at the parking lot of the Bear Valley Visitor Center, near the restrooms, one-half mile west of Olema on Bear Valley Road. Signs clearly point the way. Always open. Admission: free. Phone: (415) 663-1092.

Ever feel a pressing need to put one foot on the North American plate and the other on the Pacific plate, to straddle the fault line as two massive pieces of the earth grind past each other? Here's your chance to do some "tectonic surfing." The Earthquake Trail is right on top of the San Andreas fault for part of its length, with signs indicating exactly where. You can even see a fence that has shifted 16 feet—which isn't surprising when you remember that this very spot was the epicenter of the 1906 quake.

PACIFICA

Pacific Coast Fog Festival: fourth weekend in September. On Palmetto Avenue, between Shell and Salada Streets. From Highway 1, take the Paloma Avenue exit.

For more information, call (415) 346-4446 or (415) 875-7335.

People in Pacifica, sick of their town's reputation as a fogbound drearsville, instigated the Fog Capital of the West Contest. Weather forecasters all over the Pacific Coast nominate their own cities, citing the texture and qualities of the fog itself, shipwreck statistics, fog-related legends, and the like. A team of meteorologists decides the winner and announces it at the Fog Fest, where they award the winning weatherperson a waterproof trench-coat. Pacifica seldom wins its own contest. In fact, for the last few years the city has had to rent a fog machine to give the festival an appropriately damp ambience.

PALO ALTO

Barbie Doll Hall of Fame: in the Doll Studio, 325 Hamilton Avenue (between Bryant and Waverly), just a few blocks north of the Stanford University campus. Open Tuesday–Friday, 1:30–4 P.M., Saturday, 10:30 A.M.–12:30 P.M. Admission: $2; children, $1; children under 5, free. Phone: (415) 326-5841.

Threw out your Barbie collection when you got your first boyfriend? Feel like a fool? Have a tearful reunion with Malibu Barbie; Growing-Up Skipper; and ever-faithful Ken, the Ned Nickerson of the doll kingdom, at this remarkable plastic menagerie. Over 8,000 dolls are on display—dating back to Barbie's torpedo-breasted, wasp-waisted, ponytailed debut in 1959. America's mutating fashions and values will make you chuckle and gasp as you inspect the myriad costumes the dolls are wearing (remember that tiny nylon pantsuit you cajoled Mom into buying back in 1971?). Added bonus: Barbie's dreamhouse, through the ages.

San Andreas Fault Trail: in Los Trancos Open Space Preserve; in Palo Alto city limits, but south of Stanford University campus. Take Page Mill Road south from Palo Alto and Highway 280 six winding miles; you'll see the Los Trancos parking lot on your right. The trail leads from the parking lot and is clearly marked. Open daylight hours. Admission: free. Phone: (415) 949-5500.

Pick up a brochure at the first stop of this classy earthquake trail and follow the 13 stops to earthquake nirvana. See "sag ponds," rifts, cracks in the earth, fault line springs, trees knocked over in 1906, and yellow-banded posts that mark the exact location of the San Andreas fault. Note that the required displaced fence is actually *simulated,* built to show what it would have looked like *if* an earthquake had shifted it. Awww—we want the real thing.

PORT COSTA
(Two miles east of Crockett)

Pinhead Last Supper: in Muriel's Dollhouse Museum, 33 Canyon Lake Drive, near the Carquinez Strait. Open Tuesday–Sunday, 10 A.M.–7 P.M. Admission: $1; children under 13, 25¢. Phone: (415) 787-2820.

We couldn't tell you how many angels can dance on the head of a pin, but we do know how many apostles can *sit* on the head of a pin: 12, plus one Messiah thrown in for good measure. Generally we shy away from doll museums as being too common and too cutesy, but this particular museum has—in addition to its dolls, dollhouses, and dioramas—one astounding curiosity made by Ecuadorian painter Manual Andrada, who plucks hairs from the backs of his hands and with them paints the world's tiniest miniatures. This microscopic version of Leonardo's "Last Supper" is no bigger than one of the grains of salt spilled by Judas in the original.

Rocket Ships and Trojan Horses: on Carquinez Scenic Drive, one-quarter mile west of its intersection with Canyon Lake Drive; the first house you see as you approach Port Costa from Crockett, on the north side of the road. Visible anytime. Admission: free.

"Earth to Port Costa. Earth to Port Costa. Blast off in five minutes!" The 15-foot gleaming metal rocket ship in Clayton Bailey's yard shoots flames out the back sometimes at night, blasting off to points unknown. Every morning it's back in the yard, secret mission accomplished. Keeping the rocket company is a jet-powered whirligig car, its missing lower half severely limiting its mobility. Up on the hill to the northwest of the rocket, a pair of horses graze peacefully, quietly, unmovingly—in fact, a little *too* unmovingly. They're actually flat wooden horse sculptures (dubbed "The Trojan Horses") put there by another of the wily Bailey clan "to startle and amaze passersby." Plans are afoot at the Bailey house to install even more elaborate gadgetry in the yard.

SAN FRANCISCO

Blessing of the Fleet: first Sunday in October. Procession begins at 2 P.M. in front of Sts. Peter and Paul Church, 666 Filbert Street, facing Washington Square Park in North Beach, and continues down Columbus Street to Jefferson Street, Fisherman's Wharf, and finally to Pier 45. For more information, call (415) 421-0809.

San Franciscans of Sicilian descent hold the Madonna del Lume (Madonna of the Candle) in special regard. She's the traditional patroness of fishermen, and Sicilians' lives are forever linked with the sea. A statue of the Madonna is carried along the procession route, and at the water's edge, a North Beach priest blesses the fishing fleet. This San Francisco tradition is well over 50 years old.

Cable Car Museum: 1202 Mason Street, at Washington Street, in the Cable Car Barn. Open daily in summer, 10 A.M.–6 P.M.; daily in winter, 10 A.M.–5 P.M. Admission: free. Phone: (415) 474-1887.

Can't afford to ride the cable cars? Neither can we. But you can learn about 'em here. This mostly historical museum features old cable cars, samples of worn-out cables and broken brakes, pictures, models, letters, and other memorabilia. The museum overlooks the big turbine that operates the cable that drives the cars. Sit on a bench and watch the thick cables humming and spinning. It's positively hypnotic.

Camera Obscura: at Cliff House, far western tip of San Francisco, at the west end of Point Lobos Avenue. Camera Obscura is behind the Cliff House, on the lower terrace. Open daily, 10 A.M.–4 P.M. Admission: $1; children, 50¢. Phone: (415) 387-5693.

The scenery glitters and undulates—like a living movie—across the plywood screen. This camera obscura has been here 40 years, and was initially installed by the owner of the now-defunct amusement park, Playland by the Sea. It's housed in a building that resembles a camera.

Canticle of the Sun: in Duquette Pavilion, 1839 Geary Boulevard, at Fillmore Street. Open Wednesday–Sunday, 11 A.M.–4 P.M. Admission: $4; seniors and students, $2; children under 12, free. Phone: (415) 563-7321.

Is it heaven? Twenty-five-foot archangels loom all around you, paradisiacal in amethyst, seashells, and peacock feathers; weird towers and totem poles echo with starry music; suns, moons, masks, and wheels twirl and flash. Longtime artist and set designer Tony Duquette's "celebrational environment" in honor of St. Francis—the city's patron saint—is part shrine, part giant's jewel-box. Duquette's love for the angels and saints is mixed with an almost-pagan delight in the living world: His Archangel Ariel, "Lord of winds and the green earth," is festooned with malachite, copper, and fake emeralds. Sprawling, glittering 18-by-20-foot tapestries depict animals, fish, insects, seaweed....

Carousel Museum: 633 Beach Street, at Hyde Street, across the street from The Cannery. Open daily in summer, 10 A.M.–6 P.M.; daily in winter, 10 A.M.–5 P.M. Admission: $2; seniors, $1; children under 12, free. Phone: (415) 928-0550.

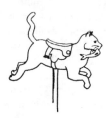

When you were little and you rode the carousel, you didn't know it was art, didja? Well, now you know. Each of the museum's meticulously carved animals has a personality all its own. Along with a valiant fish-tailed horse, you'll see a carousel fish, ostrich, goat, St. Bernard, camel, bear, pigs, and more. A studio in the museum allows you to watch craftspeople restoring animals. Note the rows of spare tails on the wall.

Cartoon Art Museum: 665 3rd Street, Room 505, fifth floor, near Townsend Street. Open Thursday and Friday, noon–6 P.M.; Saturday, 10 A.M.–4 P.M. Admission: $1; children under 12, 50¢. Phone: (415) 546-3922.

Original sketches by renowned cartoonists reveal the skill and detail that go into a good cartoon, and will resoundingly convince you never again to take cartoons for granted. Comic books are also on display here, as are cartoon-character dolls and toys: Mighty Mouse, Superman, Woody Woodpecker, and the like. We say it's high time somebody put Daffy Duck on a par with Michelangelo's David, dagnabbit.

Chinese Historical Society Museum: 17 Jack Kerouac Street (formerly Adler Place), between Grant and

Columbus Avenues, at the northern edge of Chinatown. Open Tuesday–Saturday, 1–5 P.M. Admission: free. Phone: (415) 391-1188.

The Chinese immigrant experience—seldom discussed in public schools—is traced in a variety of exhibits. Most striking are a long queue (man's braid), cut off long ago; a joss-house altar from a now-destroyed temple in Napa; and instruments from the office of Dr. Li Po Tai, an herbalist operating in 19th-century San Francisco's Chinatown. Among the more painful exhibits are "Persecution," "The Secluded Ghetto," and "Angel Island Interrogations."

Coltrane Church: 351 Divisadero Street, between Oak Street and Page Street. Services on Sunday at 11:45 A.M. and 6 P.M., and on Wednesday evenings. Phone: (415) 621-4054.

Some musicians spawn fan clubs; others have "cult followings." Only John Coltrane is a religion unto himself. The legendary jazz saxophonist is admired everywhere as one of the great musicians and improvisors of all time. Here in San Francisco, followers have dared to take the leap from admiration to worship. Services in the church (whose official name is "One Mind Temple Evolutionary Transitional Church of Christ, St. John Coltrane Memorial Branch") incorporate Coltrane's music into the proceedings. Wednesday and Sunday nights are free jazz and bop jam sessions. Gabriel just ain't hip enough.

Commedia Bowl: on the Sunday before Super Bowl Sunday, sometime in mid-January. At Galileo High School football field, 1055 Bay Street at Van Ness Avenue. Kickoff time around noon. Admission: $5 (usually). For more information, call (415) 285-2727 (BUL-CRAP).

America's most cherished ritual—the Super Bowl—is put through the comic meat-grinder in the season's zaniest football game. Comedy troupe Fratelli Bologna faces off against the Wonderteam, composed of various local funnymen and lunatics. Nothing is sacred: Footballs explode, plays are run backward, teams wear their undershorts on the outside, and players compete in rubber masks and Bigfoot costumes. In past games, the Bolognas played one quarter on stilts, and had Mayor Art Agnos as a running back. A few years ago the referees actually outscored one of the teams and came in second. Who needs the NFL?

Festival of the Chariots: on a Sunday sometime between August 14 and 28; starts at noon at Fell Street and Stanyan Street and continues on John F. Kennedy Drive through Golden Gate Park to Marx Meadow. For exact date and more information, call (415) 647-3037.

The Jews have Passover, the Christians have Christmas, and the witches have Beltane—but what do the Hare Krishnas have to break up the monotony of asking for spare change? They've got the Festival of the Chariots, the reddest red-letter day on the Krishna Kalendar. A towering colorful Juggernaut—a replica of the original in Benares, India—rumbles its way through Golden Gate Park, to the sounds of clanging finger cymbals and a thousand devout chanters. An allegorical Krishna play in Marx Meadow caps off the festivities.

Golden Gate Fortune Cookie Company: 56 Ross Alley, between Jackson Street and Washington Street, just west of Grant Avenue, in Chinatown. Open daily, 9 A.M.–9 P.M. Admission: free. Phone: (415) 781-3956.

The cookies come out of a machine, limp and flat. Workers insert the printed fortunes and fold the cookies by hand, one by one. Old-fashioned, eh? Well, what about that sign in the window announcing that this is the home of "French Adult Fortune Cookies"? Yup, and they're printed on saucy yellow paper—in Chinese tradition, yellow represents nastiness. Our investigations revealed: "Fu Ling Yu says: Zombie is something some men drink and other men marry." And: "Smart girl is one who play post office all night and get no mail in box."

Gregorian Chant: Ancient Tridentine Catholic Church, 130 11th Avenue, between California and Lake Streets. On Sundays at 9:30 A.M. For more information, call (415) 585-2404 or (415) 751-0066.

Remember how it was a few hundred years ago, when you could hear bell-like reverent harmonies echoing over every monastery wall? These days it's hard to find a real Gregorian chant, but this church keeps up the tradition. Sunday Mass is accompanied by a full choir singing the chants—it's music so rich and textured you'll want to touch it.

The Guinness Museum of World Records: 235 Jefferson Street, at Fisherman's Wharf. Open in summer, Sunday–Thursday, 9 A.M.–11 P.M.; Friday and Saturday, 9 A.M.–midnight; in winter, Sunday–Thursday, 10 A.M.–11 P.M.; Friday and Saturday, 10 A.M.–midnight. Admission: $5.95; students, $4.75; children 5–12, $2.75; children under 5, free. Phone: (415) 771-9890.

We know, we know, it's a goofy tourist trap. Still, any museum that focuses on the extremes of the human experience can't help but be unusual, no matter how overpackaged and overpriced. This is basically a walk-through version of the *Guinness Book of World Records*, with the same emphasis on tiny things, huge things, fast things, and eccentric people.

Haight-Ashbury Homes of the Stars: During the 1960s, the Haight-Ashbury district was home to what seemed like 90 percent of the world's supply of hippies. But the area also was home to many legendary characters, the most famous—and notorious—being The Grateful Dead, Jefferson Airplane, and the Manson family. For those of you who can't go home without a picture of yourself in front of the former residence of some near-mythic character, we provide their addresses.

The Grateful Dead: 710 Ashbury Street between Waller Street and Frederick Street.
This grayish-green three-story Victorian shows no hint of its secret past life as the headquarters of the wildest band of the 1960s.
The Manson family: 636 Cole Street, between Haight Street and Waller Street.
Charles Manson lived in a lot of places; this grim beige duplex was only one of his stops on the road to infamy.
Jefferson Airplane: 2400 Fulton Street, at Willard Street North.
Once a cultural focal point, this white Georgian mansion (now guarded by a video camera security system) is still headquarters to the current incarnation of Jefferson Airplane.

* * * *

Kong Chow Temple: 855 Stockton Street, fourth floor, in Chinatown. Open daily, 9 A.M.–4 P.M. Admission: free.

The air is intoxicatingly thick with incense in this ornate temple, where thousands of crimson strips of paper waft in the breeze. Carved wooden decorations and deities—including the god Kwan Ti—are dizzyingly intricate; another treasure is a huge antique bell. Best of all, near the door, is a relic from a visit paid here by Mrs. Harry Truman in June 1948. She asked the oracle whether her husband would win the upcoming election: On display here is a copy of the affirmative reply.

Lotus Fortune Cookie Company: 14 Otis Street, near Mission Street and South Van Ness Avenue. Open Monday–Friday, 8 A.M.–5:30 P.M. (Before wandering around the factory, ask permission in the office, just to the right of the entrance.) Admission: free. Phone: (415) 552-0759.

Steaming mugs of tea stand waiting for the workers to drink, but the most interesting workers in this rather high-tech factory are the machines, not the humans. One machine squirts dollops of golden batter into round flat molds, then presses and cooks them. The best machine of all grabs the soft cookies one by one, shoves a fortune into each one with alarming savagery, then folds the cookie and sends it on its way.

Lotus Garden Temple: 532 Grant Avenue (upstairs), inside the Lotus Garden Restaurant, in Chinatown. Open Tuesday–Sunday, 10 A.M.–6 P.M. Admission: free. Phone: (415) 433-2623.

Food offerings, artfully arranged, line the altars: melons, steamed rice, plump pastries, vegetables, beans, perfect apples and oranges. Along one wall are photographs of deceased loved ones. And overhead, a relic from a time when this was not yet a Taoist temple: a great old stained-glass sunroof.

Museum of Modern Mythology: 693 Mission Street, at Third Street, on the ninth floor. Open Thursday–Saturday, noon–5 P.M. Admission: $2; children, 50¢. Phone: (415) 546-0202.

Chiquita Banana, Mr. Peanut, The Jolly Green Giant, Cap'n Crunch: Like characters in any myth, they're aggressive, intense message-bearers. And if shopping is our culture's main ritual, then these critters just might be deities. That's the concept here at the museum, where (in addition to changing exhibits, such as a recent one on polyester shirts) you can reunite with stuffed Quisp dolls, a nodding-headed plastic Colonel Sanders, and the like. A typed sheet provides background on each.

Museum of the Money of the American West: 400 California Street, in the Bank of California. Go to the left as you enter, downstairs to the basement. Open Monday–Thursday, 10 A.M.–3:30 P.M.; Friday, 10 A.M.–5 P.M. Admission: free. Phone: (415) 765-3174.

Next time you're at a swanky San Francisco cocktail party, being humiliated by urbane sophisticates who treat you like a bumpkin for not knowing any City trivia, spring this question on 'em: Where in San Francisco can you find a $3 bill personally signed by Brigham Young? Only you will know that the answer is the Museum of the Money of the American West, wherein you'll see, besides the extremely rare 1849 State of Deseret Mormon currency, Gold Rush-era coins bearing the motto "In Gold We Trust"; gargantuan nuggets from the Mother Lode; $50 coins; and hyperdelicate balances used to detect gold coins hollowed out and filled with, of all things, platinum (back when platinum was cheap).

The Museum of Ophthalmology: 655 Beach Street, on the third floor, across the street from the Cannery, near the end of Columbus Avenue. Open Monday–Friday, 8 A.M.–5 P.M. Admission: free. Phone: (415) 561-8500.

Peekaboo! Sure, some of the exhibits focus on horrifying surgical tools and eye diseases, but others cover less visceral ground: collections of bejewelled antique lorgnettes and opera glasses, elegant glasses cases, and an interesting Swedish antiblindness good-luck charm. One exhibit has a great collection of glass eye cups; another has glasses worn by Nazi concentration camp victims. Most mesmerizing of all are the hand-blown glass models of diseased eyes, so realistic you'd swear some of them were watching you.

Museum of Russian Culture: 2450 Sutter Street, at Divisadero Street. Open Wednesday–Saturday, 11 A.M.–3 P.M. Admission: free. Phone: (415) 921-4082.

That's not Soviet; that's Russian—as white as the snows over St. Petersburg. Dusty, cheek-by-jowl exhibits here sing a sad song of nostalgia for the days of the czar: old Russian jewelry, silverware, portraits of the czar's ill-fated family; innumerable rich and melancholy trinkets line the tables and shelves like so many Communists in line for their sugar rations. Honor is given to famous Americans of Russian descent, like Natalie Wood (née Natasha Gurdin). Most poignant of all is a cigarette butt once tossed away by Czar Nicholas—now mounted and lovingly framed.

Near Escapes Tours: call (415) 921-1392 or write to P.O. Box 3005, San Francisco, CA 94119, to find out about current tours and times and to make reservations. Tour prices range from $20–$65.

Near Escapes is a tour company that caters to the kind of people that buy books like *America Off the Wall*. Many of their special theme tours go where motivated tourists couldn't go even if they wanted to. A recent newsletter lists trips underneath the Santa Cruz Boardwalk to see the subterranean workings, behind-the-scenes glimpses of Steinhart Aquarium and Chinatown, rides in rocketing Grand Prix race cars, and the ever-popular tour of Colma cemeteries.

Norras Temple: 109 Waverly Place, between Clay and Washington Streets, just west of Grant Avenue, in Chinatown. Open daily, 9 A.M.–3 P.M. Admission: free. Phone: (415) 362-1993.

Here's another for your Chinese-temples-at-the-top-of-killer-staircases agenda. Every other Sunday, monks are on the premises, and if you're polite and respectful, you can watch them going about their duties.

Oasis Pool Parties: 11th Street and Folsom Street, south of Market. Pool open on Friday, noon–7 P.M., and Sunday, noon–2 A.M. Admission: free (but you must be over 21). Phone: (415) 621-8119.

Mild-mannered dance club five days a week, the Oasis becomes a pool party paradise on Fridays and Sundays. The dance floor is a clear plexiglass pool cover; take it off, and jump into the fun-filled pool! Beach balls and inflatable toys abound as revelers trade in their dancing shoes for bikinis and backstroke to the pounding beat laid down by the in-house DJ. C'mon everybody—do The Swim!

Ripley's Believe It or Not! Museum: 175 Jefferson Street, at Fisherman's Wharf. Open Sunday–Thursday, 10 A.M.–10 P.M.; Friday and Saturday, 10 A.M.–midnight. Admission: $5.95; children 13–17, $4.75; children 5–12, $2.75; children under 5, free. Phone: (415) 771-6188.

This is one of the first Ripley's museums—and still just about the best. Among the highlights are scores of truly amazing miniatures, art and sculpture made from jellybeans and toothpicks, and a series of stores that sell some remarkably weird curios. Other Ripley's museums rely too heavily on wax figures and *representations* of oddities; the real stuff is here. Out front is the "World's Most Lifelike Statue," a full-body self-portrait that incorporates the artist's own hair and nails. Despite a well-placed loincloth, you can still catch a glimpse of his you-know-what from the back as he rotates.

St. Stupid's Day Parade: on April 1, starting at noon. If April 1 is a weekday, the parade starts at Justin Herman Plaza at the foot of Market Street (near its intersection with Steuart Street) and zigzags through the financial district, up Market to California Street, to Battery Street and beyond. If April 1 falls on a weekend, the parade starts at the base of the Transamerica Pyramid (Montgomery Street and Columbus Avenue) and continues straight up Columbus to Washington Square Park. For more information, call (415) 332-8744 (D FAT PIG).

April 1 is the traditional All Fooles' Day and was for centuries given over to outrageous behavior and "Fooles' Rule." The only modern remnants of this once-major celebration are the few half-hearted April Fools' practical jokes perpetrated by drunken college students. Now All Fooles' Day is back—with a slight name change. Hundreds of wackos, misfits, and professional comedians lay the financial district to satirical waste. Parade stops include the Tomb of St. Stupid, the Pacific S'ock Exchange (where socks are exchanged), and the giant bolts that keep the city from sliding into the bay. Put on a green wig, some wax lips, and join the hilarity.

Sherlock Holmes Exhibits: in the Sherlock Holmes, Esq. Lounge, in the Union Square Holiday Inn, 480 Sutter Street, at Powell Street, on the 30th floor. Exhibits are to your right as you enter the bar. Open daily, 4 P.M.–1 A.M. Admission: free. For more information, call (415) 398-8900.

Holmes and Watson—interrupted by a client in distress—just ran out the door, leaving their flat alone, exposed, and free for us to examine at our leisure. Behind glass at the end of a "gaslit" hallway is a life-size replica of 221B Baker Street, with all the details: a chemistry set in one corner, Holmes' purple dressing gown, a whippet-headed cane. On the table is a half-eaten meal: a meat pie, crackers, etc. Elsewhere along the hallway are ornately framed, brilliantly arranged little collections of "clues": in one, a pair of severed ears; in another, a porcelain goose, a blue gem, and a tiny brass footlocker.

Snapshot Heaven: Alamo Square, facing east; on Steiner Street between Fulton and Hayes Streets. Always visible.

Postcards and brochures depicting San Francisco often show a row of spiffy Victorian houses on a hill, with downtown skyscrapers in the distant background. Visitors to the city spend hours wandering around, trying to find this elusive photo spot. Search no more.

Spontaneous Opera: at Caffe Trieste, 601 Vallejo Street, at Grant Avenue, in North Beach. Saturdays, 1–4 P.M. (times vary). Phone: (415) 392-6739.

The owner's son, daughter, nieces, and nephews leap into golden-throated action; somebody grabs an accordion; and arias, mingling with the tang of espresso, waft out into the streets and the fog. Saturday afternoon opera is a 30-year tradition at this most historic of North Beach cafés, where Beat poets once soaked up inspiration and scribbled great lines on rumpled napkins, and where everything's still *molto Italiano*, the way all of North Beach used to be. *Bravissimo!*

Tattoo Museum: 30 7th Street, at Market Street. Open daily, noon–6 P.M. Admission: free. Phone: (415) 864-9798.

Lyle Tuttle, one of the West's most famous needle-slingers, fills his museum with artifacts that make you realize tattoos are much more than just something drunken sailors get, late at night. A mannequin displays the all-over tattooing customs of the South Pacific; photos trace the careers of tattooed men and women; hundreds of colorful designs show the variety and intensity of tattoos. Crude but ingenious tattoo machines, handmade in prisons, employ sharpened ballpoint pens and other surprising media. Can't decide whether to take the plunge yourself? Tuttle's studio is on the premises. The sound of buzzing needles follows you everywhere.

Tin How Temple (aka Tien How): 125 Waverly Place, between Clay and Washington Streets, on the top floor, just west of Grant Avenue, in Chinatown. Open daily, 10 A.M.–4 P.M. Admission: voluntary donation.

San Francisco's oldest temple, dedicated to the Queen of Heaven, blossoms with red offertory papers; hundreds of them hang from the ceiling, as do hundreds of lanterns. Incense sticks, smoldering in alcoves, waft their smoke among the carved wooden deities; and oranges, left by the faithful as offerings, wait mutely on the altars. The temple dates back to the 1850s.

Tombstone Gutters: in Buena Vista Park, near Duboce Avenue and Buena Vista Avenue. Always visible. Admission: free. For more information, call (415) 558-3354.

In the early 1900s, San Francisco evicted all its cemeteries and sent them packing to Colma. Thousands of bodies were dumped unceremoniously into mass graves. The city was left with piles of abandoned, old marble tombstones. Feeling too spooked to use them as building material and too guilty to throw away such nice marble, the city found a compromise: Use them to pave the rain gutters along the pathways in Buena Vista Park. You have to look hard to find inscriptions (best hunting grounds are along the pathways above the tennis court at the park's northeastern end), but the thrill of finding a weathered "...his soul..." or "...1865..." is worth the effort.

Vedanta Society Temple: 2963 Webster Street, at Fillmore Street. Always visible.

This architectural gumbo may well be the Tower of Babel: Its features are borrowed from spiritual sources that span the globe. Look hard enough at this sprawling gray edifice and you'll see a Taj Mahal dome, a Saracenic crescent, an onionesque Russian Orthodox dome, iron filigree balconies, Victorian gingerbread, Moorish arches, turrets...oh yeah, and bay windows.

Vibrator Museum: at Good Vibrations, 3492 22nd Street, at Dolores Street, in the Mission District. Open Monday–Saturday, noon–6 P.M.; Sunday, 1–5 P.M. Admission: free. Phone: (415) 550-7399.

A few dozen vintage vibrators sit mutely on a shelf, the picture of nonchalance. If these vibrators were human, they'd be shuffling their feet and bleating, "Who, me?" They're green, blue, pink—one of them looks like the offspring of a doorknob and an eggbeater; another straps handily onto your wrist; still another has a scary suction cup on the end. Most have names: Marvolator, Beauty Patter, Vim (that's the one with the suction cup), Handy

Hannah. (The shop sells diverse vibrators, too, and interesting sexual self-help books.)

Wave Organ: at the tip of the Yacht Harbor Breakwater. To get there, go west on Marina Boulevard past Baker Street; turn right (north) on Yacht Road, and walk past the St. Francis Yacht Club to the end of the breakwater. Always open. Admission: free.

Pipes—extending down below the water level—emerge from the rough stonework, looking like alien periscopes spying on the Marina Green kite-flyers. But they're for listening in, not seeing out of; place your ear to any of the pipes for a soothing, gurgling aural experience. The sounds emanating from the pipes are caused by the motion of the waves below. (Extra bonus: The breakwater is made of landfill from uprooted cemeteries.)

The World of Economics: 101 Market Street, at Spear Street, in the Federal Reserve Bank lobby. Open Monday–Friday, 9 A.M.–4:30 P.M. Admission: free. Phone: (415) 974-2000.

Welcome to the wacky World of Economics! Do you know what the government does with our hard-earned $5 bills after putting them through shredding machines? They use them for firelogs and *landfill,* for god sakes. No wonder the economy's in the dumps. With weird trivia like this, clever cartoons, splashy 3-D charts, and electronic games, the World of Economics puts the fun back into capitalist indoctrination. Tired of shooting aliens and enemy tanks at your local video parlor? The free video games here will have you making policy decisions, running a muffin factory, and saving the stock market from collapse. Anybody can kill an alien; it takes a real he-man to turn a profit.

World of Oil: 555 Market Street, between 1st and 2nd Streets, in the Chevron Building, to the right as you enter. Open Monday–Friday, 9 A.M.–4 P.M. Admission: free. Phone: (415) 894-4895.

Half public affairs gimmick and half museum, World of Oil teaches no more about oil than it does about Chevron's oil philosophy. Electronic oil trivia quiz games award extra points for pro-oil exploration answers and penalize answers that smack of environmentalism. Other, less political, exhibits have microscopes to look at fossil microbes, vicious-looking rock-cutting drill bits, sophisticated electric "story of oil" displays, and a mock-up of the world's first gas station. A spoonful of sugar helps the crude oil go down....

SAN JOSE

American Museum of Quilts: 766 South 2nd Street (at East Virginia Street), just south of Highway 280 and the San Jose State University campus. Open Tuesday–Saturday, 10 A.M.–4 P.M. Admission: free, but donations are welcomed. Phone: (408) 971-0323.

Changing exhibits explore the kaleidoscopic variety found in quilts and related crafts. On any given visit, you might see Afro-American quilts, Mayan textiles, Labradorian rugs made by fishermen's wives, Amish quilts, Depression-era quilts, or contemporary quilts. You can look, but unfortunately, you can't snuggle.

Happy Hollow: 1300 Senter Road (at Story Road), in Kelley Park, east of downtown. Open Monday–Saturday, 10 A.M.–5 P.M.; Sunday, 11 A.M.–6 P.M. Admission: $2.25; children and seniors, $1.75; people under 2 and over 80, free. Phone: (408) 292-8188.

Buy your ticket in a castle, your snack in a pirate ship, your ice cream in a lighthouse...and those are just the concessions. Also here are a little haunted house, a giant walk-in shoe, a house of mirrors, a maze, a petting zoo, a crooked house, and the least ferocious Viking ship you ever saw. If you're into fantasies (and you must be, if you're reading this), don't miss the annual August snowman-building contest (call for current date): Kids turn seven tons of crushed ice into hilariously costumed characters, who ungratefully melt away with some rapidity.

Rosicrucian Egyptian Museum: at the intersection of Park and Naglee Avenues, south of the airport. Open Tuesday–Sunday, 9 A.M.–5 P.M. Admission: $3; seniors, $2.50; children 12–17, $1; children under 12, free. Phone: (408) 287-2807.

What is a notoriously secretive and esoteric religious sect doing in charge of the finest collection of mummies and Egyptian artifacts this side of Thebes? It's all part of an elaborate plan, you see, to prove once and for all that the Rosicrucians were founded by Egyptians 3,400 years ago, as claimed. Hey, if we weren't, then where'd we get all this Egyptian stuff? The collection is heaven (or, if you prefer, afterlife) for mummy-lovers, with lots of first-rate human and animal mummies and even a convincing walk-in Egyptian tomb.

Winchester Mystery House: 525 South Winchester Boulevard, between Highway 280 and Stevens Creek Boulevard. Open mid-June to Labor Day, daily, 9 A.M.– 5:30 P.M.; early June and September, Monday–Friday, 9 A.M.–4:30 P.M.; Saturday and Sunday, 9 A.M.–5 P.M.; October and March–May, Monday–Friday, 9 A.M.–4 P.M.; Saturday and Sunday, 9 A.M.–4:30 P.M.; November– February, daily, 9:30 A.M.–4 P.M. Admission: $8.95; seniors, $7.45; children 6–12, $4.95; children under 5, free. Phone: (408) 247-2101 or (408) 247-2000.

Sarah Winchester, feeling a little guilty about the $20 million she inherited from her rifle-making husband, went to a medium who informed her that half the ghosts in North America were hopping mad and out to get her. The only solution, of course, was to build additions to her house 24 hours a day every day until she died. Squadrons of carpenters toiled incessantly for 38 years, building useless stairways, sealed-off rooms, windows and doors that opened to nothing, ad infinitum. The unfinished product—160 mazelike rooms—ranks among the strangest buildings on Earth. Little is made of the fact that Winchester also manufactured roller skates.

SAN QUENTIN
(Five miles southeast of San Rafael)

Prison Handicraft Shop: at the Main Gate (east side) of San Quentin Prison. From Marin County, take Highway 580 east and get off at the last exit (marked San Quentin) before coming onto the Richmond-San Rafael Bridge. (If you're coming west off the bridge, get off at the first exit.) Follow the road until it ends at the gate. Open Wednesday–Sunday, 8 A.M.–4 P.M. Phone: (415) 454-1460.

Though its selection is not quite as extensive as that of Neiman-Marcus, the San Quentin gift shop does offer a unique selection found nowhere else: moccasins, music boxes, leatherwork, and original art made by embezzlers and murderers. Across from the shop is the prison post office; letters mailed from here are stamped "San Quentin." Great for practical joke postcards: "Dear Mary, I've had a few problems since I last wrote to you...."

SAUSALITO

California Marine Mammal Center: in the Golden Gate National Recreation Area. From San Francisco, go north over the Golden Gate Bridge, turn west on Bunker Road, continue about two miles, cross the bridge over Rodeo Lagoon, and watch for the CMMC sign. Open daily, 10 A.M.–4 P.M., for walk-through self-guided tours. Guided tours for groups on Saturday and Sunday. Admission: free. Phone: (415) 331-7325 (331-SEAL).

This is the world's wettest hospital, dedicated to saving and rehabilitating sick, injured, or stranded sea mammals. The goal is not to keep the animals but to heal them and then return them to the ocean. You can watch through a chain-link fence as the volunteer staff feeds the animals, exercises them, and administers medicine. Among the 40-odd "patients" you're likely to see are elephant seals, sea lions, dolphins, porpoises—even whales. The diseases and injuries that brought the creatures here are not pretty, but the healing atmosphere is inspiring.

San Francisco Bay and Delta Model: 2100 Bridgeway, at Marinship Way, northern part of town. Open Tuesday–Friday, 9 A.M.–4 P.M.; Saturday and Sunday, 10 A.M.–6 P.M. (closed on Sundays in winter). Admission: free. Phone: (415) 332-3871. Call ahead of time to make sure the model has water in it.

A highly detailed, scaled-down model of the entire Bay Area and Delta regions is used to predict and simulate the effect of tidal changes on the bay. Actual fresh water trickles in through the Delta, and saltwater surges in through the Golden Gate; tides rise and fall; interactions are measured; and the effects of industry and climate changes on wildlife are analyzed. The public is invited to watch the marine engineers play with their big toy. Late at night, when no one's around, they play the Polar Ice Caps Are Melting! game and drown everybody.

SUNNYVALE

Fruit Cocktail Water Tower: center of Sunnyvale Business Park, at the corner of Mathilda Avenue North and California Avenue. Always visible.

Can you loan us a can-opener? We've discovered a giant can of fruit cocktail. This 20,000-gallon water tank on its

100-foot pedestal, built in 1907, stands on the former site of the Libby fruit cannery. It's painted to represent a 1930s-era can of fruit cocktail—a delicacy, the legend goes, that was invented sort of by accident at the Sunnyvale plant. The cannery's gone but the can remains, protected like some endangered species.

SUNOL
(Five miles south of Pleasanton)

Water Temple: from Pleasanton, take Highway 680 south; get off at the Sunol exit, then turn left (south) on the Pleasanton-Sunol Road. About four-fifths of a mile down the road you will come to a four-way stop. Continue straight, through the open gates of the San Francisco Water Department. The Water Temple is straight ahead. Open Monday–Friday, 8 A.M.–4 P.M. Admission: free. For more information, call (415) 862-2233.

Nineteenth-century San Francisco had gold and good whiskey, but it had terrible water. In the 1930s, when the Water Department finally started diverting delicious water from the Sierras into the Bay Area's water supply, locals couldn't believe their good fortune. To give thanks to the generous water gods, the Water Department built this "temple": a dome-roofed, shiny-tiled, columned cement structure, Grecian in ambience. In the old days, you could stand there and watch crystal-clear mountain water gushing across the tiles, on its way to the sinks and bathtubs of San Francisco. Now, because of bureaucratic vagaries, the temple is dry as a bone. But don't hold that against it. It's still a temple.

TREASURE ISLAND
(Two miles east of San Francisco)

Treasure Island Museum: in Building 1, Treasure Island; take the Bay Bridge to the Treasure Island turnoff. The museum is in a semicircular building, the first one you see after going through the gate. Open daily, 10 A.M.–3:30 P.M. Admission: free. Phone: (415) 765-6182.

Treasure Island, now a Navy base, was originally built as the site of the 1939 Golden Gate International Exposition. The museum has two major themes: the history of the Navy, Marines, and Coast Guard in the Pacific, and memorabilia from the fair. It's the fair-related half that interests us: photographs of what was essentially an art deco fantasy city and the story behind such surprising crowd-pleasers as Sally Rand's Nude/Dude Ranch (risqué even by modern standards).

WINEHAVEN
(Three miles west of Richmond)

Ghost Town: from Richmond take Highway 580 west toward the Richmond-San Rafael Bridge; get off at the last exit before coming onto the bridge. Take Western Drive north to Point Molate U.S. Naval Fuel Depot. Always visible. Phone: (415) 234-0211.

Winehaven isn't *exactly* a ghost town. Its buildings still stand. People live there. But you won't find it on any map. It's not even a city anymore. What was once Winehaven is now Point Molate U.S. Naval Fuel Depot. Winehaven was the company town for the world's largest winery, now defunct. The huge brick wine vats on the west side of the road now hold ship fuel. The workers' houses on the hill have been taken over by Navy families. Everything in the winery has been co-opted for military purposes. Winehaven isn't dead—it's just got a serious case of amnesia.

WOODSIDE
(25 miles south of San Francisco)

Pulgas Water Temple: Five miles north of Woodside; take Canada Road north from Woodside (just west of Highway 280) past Filoli to the southern tip of Upper Crystal Springs Reservoir. From Highway 280 take the Edgewood Road exit west and turn north on Canada Road. The temple is clearly visible, and a short driveway leads to its parking lot. Always open, though occasionally the parking lot gates are closed, forcing you to park farther up Canada Road. Admission: free. For more information, call (415) 872-5900.

San Francisco's massively complicated water supply system starts on the other side of the state and ends right here at this temple, where water that has traveled hundreds of miles finally flows into the city's main reservoir. In a moment of unabashed pagan spirituality, the Water Department built this temple in gratitude to whatever deity takes credit for things like pipelines and pure water. Appropriately Greco-Roman looking, the domed temple has reverent inscriptions all around it and impressive columns. Unlike its sister temple in Sunol, you can see in this temple the travel-weary water rushing smoothly to its new home.

THE NORTH

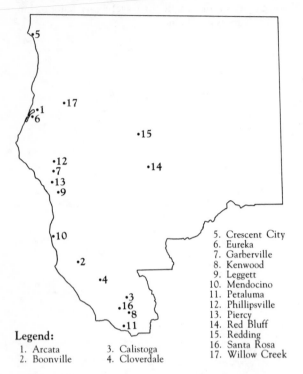

Legend:

5. Crescent City
6. Eureka
7. Garberville
8. Kenwood
9. Leggett
10. Mendocino
11. Petaluma
12. Phillipsville
13. Piercy
14. Red Bluff
15. Redding
16. Santa Rosa
17. Willow Creek

1. Arcata
2. Boonville
3. Calistoga
4. Cloverdale

California's northern shank, sparsely populated and hardly penetrated, is elegant and wild. It is the state's dense, lustrous, unbrushable mane, flowing according to its own impetuous plan.

It's odd, too. Plenty odd. All those wineries, with their spooky cellars. Yellow slugs that grow to six inches long, like gelatinous canaries. And those forests, so dark and silent: They harbor creatures not quite human, but almost—the shy, hulking Bigfoot; the wise, white-robed Lemurians rumored to dwell on Mount Shasta.

Geysers. Boiling lakes. Drive-thru trees. In the north, it's not a matter of "Where do I find the weird stuff?" Rather, it's "Can I spend the night here without the weird stuff climbing in my window and hauling me away?"

ARCATA

Annual World Championship Great Arcata-to-Ferndale Cross-Country Kinetic Sculpture Race: Memorial Day weekend (usually), starting at noon Saturday, lasting till Monday afternoon. Starting line is at Arcata Plaza, 8th and H Streets, downtown. The racecourse continues across Humboldt Bay, through Eureka, and ends on Main Street in downtown Ferndale. Spectating is free. For race information, call (707) 725-3851. For lodging/facilities information, call (800) 338-7352, or outside California, (800) 346-3482.

This is the biggie. The world championship. Three days of roads, sand dunes, seawater, mud, agony, and ecstasy. Scores of the world's most preposterous human-powered machines and mobile artworks compete "for the glory." Prizes are awarded in various categories, including First Breakdown, Mediocrity (for finishing in the middle), and Lack of Speed. The participants' and spectators' main goals are to act crazy in public and get publicity. Yet still there are always those demented few who actually try to go the fastest and look the best. Too many hormones, probably. Prime spectating points are all along the course and are often crowded. For exact route, call the above phone numbers.

ASTI
(Four miles south of Cloverdale)

Pat Paulsen Vineyards: in Asti Village, which is just a few buildings. Exit Highway 101 east to Asti, and take an immediate right turn; you can't miss it. Open daily, 10 A.M.–6 P.M. Admission: free. Phone: (707) 894-2969.

"The bouquet is simply exquisite." That sums up the typically snooty attitude you encounter at most wineries. But it's different when the winery is owned by a world-famous, not-quite-washed-up comedian. In the Asti "City Hall" (a dilapidated shack next to the tasting room), idiotic and absurd displays smack of Paulsen's deadpan humor. Garbagey thrift-store plates are labeled "Aztec serving platter" and "Pat's collection of 16th-century Venetian glass." Two paper plates with pasta glued on them recount "the Twin Semolina Miracles." The tasting room has relics of Pat's presidential campaigns.

Wine-Barrel Churches: Exit Highway 101 east to Asti and take an immediate left turn north on Frontage Road.

The churches come into view after a few hundred yards. Always visible; services on Sundays.

For decades, the only employer in the town of Asti was the Italian Swiss Colony winery. When the workers decided they needed a church, a storage hothouse was converted into a place of worship. Appropriately, the hothouse was shaped like a huge, sawed-in-half wine barrel, set on its side. In the 1950s the winery built a new church, also in the shape of a wine barrel, though the new one was larger and had a more pronounced arch. And it's made out of staves taken from old wine barrels. The church was musty and damp from the start and reeked of vino. In fact, it still smells a tad like Muscatel.

CALISTOGA

Old Faithful Geyser: 1299 Tubbs Lane, northwest end of Calistoga between Highways 128 and 29. Open in summer, daily, 9 A.M.–6 P.M.; in winter, daily 9 A.M.–5 P.M. Admission: $2.50; children 6–12, $1; children under 6, free. Phone: (707) 942-6463.

America has three regularly erupting geysers; this is the only one you have to pay to see. Every 40 minutes or so—with the emphasis on the "or so"—350-degree water spurts 60 feet in the air and cascades into a steaming pool. Hey, people go all the way to Yellowstone to see the same thing; so show a little respect, okay?

Petrified Forest: 4100 Petrified Forest Road, five miles west of town, off Highway 128. Open in summer daily, 9 A.M.–6 P.M.; in winter, daily 9 A.M.–5 P.M. Admission: $3; children under 10, free. Phone: (707) 942-6667.

If you've visited other petrified forests, you've seen the disappointing sights: "trees" that are broken up, crumbled, and a few feet long at most. Well, push that picture from your mind. These are California-style petrified trees. Some measure 120 feet long and extend another 100 feet underground. These trees are—were—giant redwoods, and these specimens are the largest petrified trees in the world. This is one of California's oldest roadside attractions: It was opened over 120 years ago.

A NATIVE TONGUE

Spain has Spanish, China has Chinese, Italy has Italian, and the town of Boonville has Boontling. The history and origins of Boontling are almost as confusing as its vocabulary. Some sources say Boontling is the only native folk language in the United States; others say there's another one, but nobody seems to know what it is. Boontling was supposedly invented by locals to bamboozle outsiders; a few residents claim it started around 1880 as a secret language between siblings. Soon the other children learned it, developed it, and used it to fool their parents. Eventually the parents caught on and shaped Boontling into a full-blown dialect. Scholars claim it is a combination of English, Scottish, and Native American Indian; most people who are familiar with it say it's nothing more than an intricate pig Latin. Though the controversy isn't exactly raging, the matter seems permanently unresolved, which is okay with Boonville residents, who generally enjoy their reputation as stubborn separatists. Several of Boontling's words are obvious contractions: *hairk* for haircut, *relf* for rail fence; *schoolch* for teacher. Others are shorthand metaphors: storms are *trashmovers*; a cocky person is a *feather leg*. Still others describe local characters: to *Charlie Ball* means to embarrass; *Tom Bacon* means mustache. But many words are absolutely inscrutable: *higs* is money; *gorm* is eat; *tidrick* is party. Boontling—called Boont for short—has all but died out as a living spoken language, but remnants of it are still around town on signs (telephone booths say "Buckey Walter" and restaurants boast "Bahl gorms") and in local phrases that tourists rarely, if ever, hear. When you're in town, stop by the Horn of Zeese Coffee Shop for a steaming-hot horn of zeese.

CLEAR LAKE

Worm Races: every Saturday in May, 11 A.M. Finals are held the last Saturday in May. Austins Park, Olympic Drive and Lakeshore Drive, on the lake, downtown. For more information, call (707) 994-3600.

Clear Lake is, say the locals, a fisherman's paradise. In a community that spends so much time brooding about night crawlers, things like worm races are bound to happen. Fifteen years ago a self-proclaimed "cousin" of Mark Twain "inherited" the writer's "genius" at "racing" unlikely animals, and the idea was born. Squeaky-clean, freshly washed worms are placed inside a three-foot circle and encouraged to get out of it. The worms, blind and legless and fatalistic, usually comply.

CLOVERDALE

Citrus Sculpture Contest: at the Citrus Fair, Presidents' Day weekend, in February. Friday–Sunday, 10 A.M.–10 P.M.; Monday, 10 A.M.–5 P.M. Main Exhibit Hall at the fairgrounds, west side of Highway 101, center of town. Admission: $3.50; children, $2. Phone: (707) 894-5790.

Let's take 90 dozen plump, glossy, vitamin-rich citrus fruits and...eat 'em? Make juice out of 'em? Send 'em to a hungry Third-World country? Naw—let's make 'em into a sculpture of a 20-foot poodle! Contestants are permitted to use other edible foods to augment the citrus in their sculptures (1,080 fruits, minimum, per sculpture). Recent entries have incorporated oatmeal, coffee grounds, and waffles. Also on display are six-by-four-foot citrus "mosaics," in which the unfortunate fruits are arstistically attached to big boards.

Grape Festival: third weekend of September. Main exhibit hall, the fairgrounds, west side of Highway 101, center of town. Admission: $2. For more information, call (707) 894-5790.

Two-man teams compete in the grape-stomping contest: One stomps grapes, barefoot, in a barrel, while the other teammate quickly scoops the resultant juice into a jug. First team to fill a jug is the winner. Winery relays feature such vinicultural fortes as bottle-corking and bottle-filling. Even teetotalers will admire the large grape "mosaics" on display and the many clever crafts made out of wine corks.

CORNING
(18 miles south of Red Bluff)

Olive Festival and Bed Race: usually the last weekend in August. Bed race begins 7 P.M., Solano and 6th Streets.

For current date and more information, call (916) 824-5550.

The beds are spartan and built for speed. But the Chamber of Commerce makes the race especially madcap by providing the riders with nightshirts and insisting that riders exchange the shirts mid-race, relay style. Another festival highlight is a guess-how-many-olives-are-in-this-big-jar contest, but how can you expect to win? These Corning folks know olives like the backs of their hands.

CRESCENT CITY

World Championship Crab Races: usually the second or third Sunday in February (varies), 10 A.M.–4 P.M. Del Norte County Fairgrounds, off Highway 101, east of downtown. Admission: $1. For current date and more information, call (707) 464-3174.

Clawed contenders clatter down a four-foot wooden racetrack, their crusty hearts pounding. Each wants so much to win for its human coach that special prize: a pair of taxidermed crabs affixed to a redwood plank. The Grand Champion has the honor of being tossed back into the sea after the race, which you have to admit is quite a piece of luck for a caught crab. Three thousand pounds' worth of the Grand Champion's nonracing friends and cousins are devoured by the hungry human sportsmen and -women at the day's end.

DOYLE
(40 miles southeast of Susanville)

Lizard Races: fourth weekend in July. Next to the community center. For more information, call (916) 827-3135.

This area abounds with bluebelly lizards and with trailers and wind. Locals collect lizards and force them to run on a track. The kids make up funny theories about how to keep their lizards from dying of the heat before the race is over. Lotsa laffs.

EUREKA

Romano Gabriel's Sculpture Garden: 315 2nd Street, between D and E Streets, in Old Town, housed in a brick structure. Technically visible anytime, but doors may occasionally be closed. For more information, call (707) 442-3738.

Romano Gabriel, late Eureka carpenter, folk artist, and Chico Marx look-alike, should have designed the whole world. We'd *really* want to live in it, then. Gabriel's front yard was the original site of the sarcastic, kaleidoscopic wooden "garden," 30 years in the making. Brave, bold trees-of-life sprout faces, fruits, and hula girls. Crimson French policemen with round mouths direct imaginary traffic. Spotted wooden sausages dangle over a deadpan sign that reads, "Italian Salami." Gabriel's people sport beards, pompadours, grimaces, nipples, and eyebrows like fuzzy caterpillars. Don't miss the chocolate-brown Calypso band.

The Stump House: 1108 Broadway (at Clark Street), west side of town. Open daily, 9 A.M.–5 P.M. Admission: free. Phone: (707) 445-2471.

In 1902, loggers felled an immense redwood, took apart 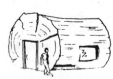 the trunk, and sent it to Eureka, where it was reassembled and hollowed out. Doors and windows were cut into it, and a tourist attraction was born. The big log measures 18 feet in diameter and is 50 feet long. (The original tree was 308 feet.) Appropriately, the Stump House now houses a redwood carving and chainsaw sculpture studio. Statues of Bigfoot and St. Francis of Assisi guard the front door.

FORT BRAGG

Stone Painting Museum: 27800 North Highway 1, seven miles north of town. Open Wednesday–Monday, 9 A.M.–4 P.M. Admission: $2; children and students, $1.25. Phone: (707) 964-9450.

Thelma Murphy Murray, a miner's granddaughter, has loved stone all her life. Thirty years ago it occurred to her that she could "paint" with stone, replacing brush stokes with bits of rock. Her pictures are part mosaic, part sculpture, part rock garden. Slivers of malachite become leaves; snowy agates become clouds. Some of Murray's works are abstract and surreal, but her own favorite is purely representational, depicting a lone cypress on Highway 1.

GARBERVILLE

Kinetic Sculpture Race: Mothers' Day. Main boulevard through town. For more information, call (707) 923-2613.

The monstrous, magnificent, human-powered machines get a trial run here in Garberville before their big race from Arcata to Ferndale. The Kinetic King and Queen preside over the hoopla, and the Kinetic Kops enforce the rules, which (among other things) state that brakes are mandatory, rum is forbidden, and the drivers' feet must never touch the ground.

GEYSERVILLE

Isis Oasis Lodge: 20889 Geyserville Avenue, south of town. Room rates: $35–$90. Phone: (707) 857-3524.

At this motel-of-the-future, you can indulge that childhood fantasy about sleeping in a tipi. And instead of a Magic Fingers machine, you get tarot readings, massage therapy, and other metaphysical ministrations. The owners are into indulging fantasies of their own: They keep bobcats, ocelots, ring-tailed servals, and an emu as pets. (The barnyard types among you will appreciate the geese, swans, sheep, and peacocks.) Tipis are available only in summer; Afghani-style canvas yurts are yours all year 'round. And the Wine-Barrel Room really is a barrel: 12 feet across, with an eight-foot domed roof.

KENWOOD

Smothers Brothers Winery: corner of Highway 12 and Warm Springs Road. Open daily, 10 A.M.–4:30 P.M. Phone: (707) 833-1010.

Mom's Favorite Red and Mom's Favorite White are popular products here. The gift shop stocks corkscrews with the brothers' pictures on them and has on display some of Tommy's gold records. Plans are underway for a big yo-yo exhibit.

World Championship Pillow Fights: July 4. Plaza Park, on Warm Springs Road. For more information, call (707) 833-2440.

No need to bring your own pillow. The local fire department provides them—that is, after they've dammed up the creek and turned it into a muddy wallow and laid a pole across the top. Competitors crawl out onto the pole, pillows in hand, and swat each other until one or both topple into the ooze.

KLAMATH
(17 miles south of Crescent City)

Tour-Thru Tree: on the north side of the Klamath River. Take the Terwer Valley exit from Highway 101; go east on Highway 169 for one-quarter mile to the tollbooth entrance, across the street from the Mobil station. Open daily, daylight hours. Admission: $1 per car; 25¢ for pedestrians and bicyclists. Phone: (707) 482-5971.

The hole through this giant redwood was cut wide enough to accommodate American cars. As a result, the remaining sides, which are supposed to hold up the tree, are disconcertingly thin. The owners compensate for this unexpected scare by providing, for your viewing pleasure, a flock of emus in a field across the road from the entrance.

Trees of Mystery: east side of Highway 101, five miles north of town. Open in summer, daily, 7:30 A.M.–8:30 P.M.; in winter, daily, daylight hours. Admission: $5; children, $2.50. Phone: (707) 482-5613.

Mother Nature made some funny trees. Human beings came along and made a tourist attraction. Funny trees here include the Cathedral (nine redwoods growing in a tight, chapel-like semicircle) and the Upside-Down Tree, whose roots reach for the sun. Along Paul Bunyan's Trail of Tall Tales, a series of man-made redwood carvings is accompanied by a kitschy taped narrative. In front of Trees of Mystery is a 49-foot Paul Bunyan (how'd he get here from Minnesota? Hitchhike?), slathering at the thought of chain-sawing the Cathedral.

LEGGETT

Chandelier Drive-Thru Tree Park: Take the Drive-Thru Tree Road exit west off Highway 101, just south of where it is joined by Highway 1; the road leads right to the park entrance. Open daily, 9 A.M.–dusk. Admission: $2.50 per car. Phone: (707) 925-6464.

Even if it didn't have a hole through it, a hole more than big enough to accommodate your Cadillac, the Chandelier Tree would still be one of the largest, oldest, and most impressive coastal redwoods in the whole region. The sign above the drive-thru passageway reads, "Since 400 B.C." We assume they mean the tree, not the hole.

MENDOCINO

Festival of the Sea: usually the first Saturday in August, 1 P.M. Ford House, Main Street, downtown. For more information, call (707) 864-3153.

Mendocino honors its deep, blue neighbor with a salty menu of seaweed recipes: Japanese miso soup, seaweed-wrapped sushi, even seaweed chips manufactured by a local seaweed harvesting company. Also on the program are Polynesian dancing demonstrations and other oceanic delights.

Pygmy Forest: three miles south of town along Highway 1, in Van Damme State Park, at Little River. Once there, you can either park at the entrance to Van Damme and hike four miles to the Pygmy Forest, or (much easier) drive one-half mile south past the park entrance, turn left (east) on Airport Road, and continue 3½ miles to the Pygmy Forest parking area, next to the well-marked hiking trail. Always open. Admission: free. Phone: (707) 937-5855.

"As you go along this stretch of the trail, imagine that you are six inches tall and looking up at this forest on each side of you. Or imagine yourself a giant, striding along above the treetops!" So commandeth the Pygmy Forest brochure. Whatever you do, don't imagine yourself five foot ten, walking through a cluster of the world's smallest trees. You might not be able to handle the reality of it all. The soil here is the most acidic and has the least amount of nutrients of any soil known; consequently, any trees stupid enough to grow here are lucky if they get to be three feet tall, even when fully grown. Many are only a foot high or even less, though they would grow to over 100 feet in normal soil. For Pygmy Forest fanatics, there's another of these "biological slums" five miles north of Mendocino in Jughandle State Reserve, in an unmarked area on the highest terrace.

MINERAL
(40 miles east of Red Bluff)

Bumpass Hell: 13 miles north of Mineral on Highway 89, about five miles north of the entrance station of Lassen Volcanic National Park. Bumpass Hell is on the right side on the road at Marker 17; signs from here indicate the trail. The Sulphur Works are one mile north of the entrance station, on the left side of the road at Marker 5. Open daily, weather permitting, which is generally June–October. Admission to Lassen Volcanic Park: $5 per vehicle. Phone: (916) 595-4444.

"**D**ouble, double, toil and trouble; in the caldron boil and bubble," the earth seems to be chanting, as it stirs up big burbling vats of foul-smelling mud and steaming pools. Its name at first appears fittingly descriptive, but Bumpass Hell is actually named after its discoverer, Kendall Vanhook Bumpass (pronounced "bumpus"). The "Hell" part applies, as the three-mile trail winds past steam geysers, boiling lakes, mud pots, fumaroles, and hot springs amid yellowish sulphurous fumes. Don't step off the walkway unless you want to sink into a boiling pool and burn your leg off—which is what happened to Bumpass. The Sulphur Works is a smaller version of the same thing a few miles back on the road.

MONTE RIO
(25 miles west of Santa Rosa)

Slug Festival: usually the third Sunday in March. Northwood Restaurant, River Road. For current date and more information, call (707) 887-1362 or (707) 575-1191.

Slugballs and slug burritos are among the delicacies dished up at the annual, and visceral, slug-off. All recipes must contain the real thing. It'll be a long time before festival-goers forget "s-lime jello," lime gelatin with a slug suspended in its emerald depths. Or the slug martini, which boasts not an olive, not a slug, but a *piece* of a slug. That's hardcore. Local politicians form the tasting panel; newspapers in Japan and Australia pick up the story. At day's end a cape and crown are placed on Superslug, the festival's mascot—usually a hefty half-pounder found in the woods nearby.

MOUNT SHASTA
(36 miles south of Yreka)

Alpenfest and Teddy Bear Festival: first weekend in February. Snow sculpture contest Saturday morning at the Ski Park; Teddy Bear Parade Saturday, noon, starting at Mt. Shasta Shopping Center. Yodel-off Sunday, 4 P.M., City Park. For more information, call (916) 926-4865.

No, you're not missing the point. There's absolutely no connection among teddy bears, yodeling, and snow sculptures. The mysterious inspiration behind this festival is just something you have to accept on faith, like the Holy Trinity. Some of the finest yodeling this side of the Matterhorn echoes through the city on Sunday. Rudimentary snowmen are simply not acceptable at the snow sculpture contest; you're much more likely to see samurai warriors and Volkswagens. And the teddy bears? They're everywhere, in every store, filling the streets, staring at you with empty eyes.

MYERS FLAT
(14 miles north of Garberville)

Shrine Drive-Thru Tree Park: Take the Myers Flat exit west off Highway 101; continue north for less than a mile on Avenue of the Giants. The entrance will be on your left (west) and is well marked. Open daily, daylight hours. Admission: $1. Phone: (707) 943-3442.

This is the undisputed original drive-thru tree. It was hollowed out by fire hundreds of years before cars were even invented; it became a tourist attraction as soon as the first road was built through the area. Nearby, in the same park, there are also a Drive-On Log, a Walk-Thru Stump, and a Hollow Log. What more could you ask for?

ORICK
(35 miles south of Crescent City)

Slug Derby: third Saturday in August, 12:45 P.M. Picnic area, Prairie Creek Redwoods State Park, north of Orick on Highway 101. For more information, call (707) 488-2171.

This is one of the granddaddies of slug events. All week, beefy banana slugs are collected in the forest. On race day, contestants select slugs from the "corral," place them inside the six-inch bull's-eye, and then yell at them.

Compassionate jockeys and park staff repeatedly spray the slugs with water during the course of the day to keep them from dying. After the race, the slugs go home to the woods, and the humans take home slug-shaped plaques.

OROVILLE

Chinese Temple: 1500 Broderick Street, south of the levee. Open Tuesday–Wednesday, 1–4 P.M.; Thursday–Monday, 11 A.M.–4:30 P.M. Admission: $1.50; children under 12, free. Phone: (916) 538-2496.

The upstairs Buddhist temple is still a place of worship—just as it has been since 1860, when the temple was built. In Oroville's heyday, the neighborhood also boasted a Chinese Opera house. This was, unfortunately, destroyed in a 1907 flood, but your tour guide can show you old opera costumes and props that were saved from oblivion.

PETALUMA

Bubbling Well Pet Memorial Park: 2462 Atlas Peak Road. Go north from Napa on Highway 121; turn left toward Silverado Country Club on Atlas Peak Road. Continue past the country club all the way up the hill. Pet Cemetery is always visible. Office open Monday–Friday, 8 A.M.–4:30 P.M.; Saturday–Sunday, 9 A.M.–4 P.M. Admission: free. Phone: (707) 255-3456.

If you've seen Errol Morris' hilarious documentary, *Gates of Heaven*, you'll recognize Bubbling Well as the setting for most of the film. Bubbling Well is the Forest Lawn of pet cemeteries, stunningly landscaped and located, with burial areas such as the Garden of Companionship, the Mermaid Pool, the St. Francis Garden, the Foothill Garden and the Olive Tree Garden. Each has its own theme. Thousands of graves in the five-acre cemetery sport statuary and inscriptions ranging from the humorous to the heart-wrenching. You know, pets are people too.

Ice Cream Museum: 824 Petaluma Boulevard, south end of downtown. Open daily, 11 A.M.–6 P.M. Admission: free. Phone: (707) 778-6008.

The many uses of fudge ripple? Cherry vanilla throughout history? Sherbet between the wars? Photos of Maurice Chevalier eating French vanilla? We wish. Still, on display at this small museum you can see antique ice-cream implements: scoops, molds, spoons, even a vintage ice-cream freezer. All are relics of an innocent time when chocolate, vanilla, and strawberry were enough.

Winners' Circle Ranch: 5911 Lakeville Highway, 5½ miles southeast of town. Open June–October, Wednesday–Sunday, 10:30 A.M.–4 P.M. Two shows per day: 11 A.M. and 2 P.M. Admission: $5; seniors and children under 12, $3. Phone: (707) 762-1808.

The "winners" in this circle are miniature horses, 34 inches high at the shoulder blades, so cute and demure that if they didn't poop, you'd swear they were toys. This breed was first developed in Europe in days of yore. During the 35-minute shows, the tiny nags display their tricks, while the ranchers provide a history of these equine curiosities that rub elbows with Fido yet share genes with National Velvet.

World Wristwrestling Championships: second Saturday in October, Veterans' Memorial Building, 1094 Petaluma Boulevard South, in the main part of town. Elimination bouts start at 1:30 P.M.; finals start at 7 P.M. Admission for the whole day: $10. Phone: (707) 778-0210.

Pure brute strength—that's what we like to see. Forget about finesse, talent, or cuteness. Petaluma may no longer be the Chicken Capital of the World, but every October it becomes the Bulging Bicep Capital of the Universe, as thick-armed men and women from all over the country grunt and grimace and slam each other to the table. A quick way to end your tennis career is to swagger into a Petaluma bar after the finals and announce, flexing your right arm, "I didn't compete this year because I wanted to give you guys a chance."

PHILLIPSVILLE
(Nine miles north of Garberville)

Chimney Tree and Hobbiton, USA: 1½ miles south of Phillipsville on the east side of the Avenue of the Giants; 7½ miles north of Garberville. Open May–September, daily, 8 A.M.–8 P.M. Admission to Hobbiton, USA: $2.50; children 3–14, $1.50; children under 3, free. Admission to Chimney Tree: free. Phone: (707) 923-2265.

The Chimney Tree is completely hollow, but still living. Its top was knocked off in a storm long ago. Hunters used to build their campfires inside, letting the smoke drift out the top. The other half of this double-whammy attraction is Hobbiton, USA, a half-mile trail through the fantasy world of J. R. R. Tolkein, complete with statuary vignettes of *Hobbit* and *Lord of the Rings* scenes and taped narrations telling the tale of Bilbo Baggins. Whether you spend your evenings locked in your motel room, speed-reading fantasy novels, or striding half-naked through groves of sequoias, this stop is sure to please.

One-Log House: on the Avenue of the Giants, center of Phillipsville (such as it is), across the street from the Madrona Motel. Open April–September, daily, 8 A.M.–7 P.M., but hours may vary. Admission: 50¢; children under 16, free. Phone: (707) 943-3688.

Two men spent eight months, in 1946, hollowing out a 32-foot redwood log, filling it with furniture, and mounting it on wheels like a mobile home. They lugged it around the country as a traveling sideshow curiosity. After a long journey it has ended up here, with all its furniture still intact. Sadly, no one has ever lived in it.

PIERCY
(Ten miles south of Garberville)

Confusion Hill: six miles south of Piercy (which isn't much of a town anyway), one-quarter mile north of the World Famous Treehouse, on the east side of Highway 101. Many signs announce it; you can't miss it. Open daily, daylight hours. Admission to Confusion Hill: $2.50; children 5–12, $1.25; children under 5, free. Admission to train ride: $2.50; children 2–12, $1.25; children under 2, free. Phone: (707) 925-6456.

This is the least publicized mystery spot in the West. No one pays it much mind, which is sad, considering that the optical illusions here are no less impressive than those in Santa Cruz or Gold Hill. Water flows uphill; people's height changes depending on where they stand; a Mystery Shack makes you lean at crazy angles. Next to Confusion Hill is the Miniature Train, which takes you on a 15-minute ride through a redwood tree trunk and past the Octopus Tree and the Smokestack Tree. Out front is a giant shoe built of redwood bark. What's the connection between these three attractions? Well, why do you think they call it Confusion Hill?

Viking Ship: 2½ miles north of Piercy, 7½ miles south of Garberville, ½ mile south of Richardson Grove on the east side of Highway 101, at the Old Grandfather Tree gift shop. Visible daily, daylight hours. Admission: free.

Scholars generally agree that the Vikings discovered North America, yet few of them realize that the Vikings got this far west. A local craftsman built this 30-foot-long, totally seaworthy ship, using redwood, memory, and imagination. The ship's dragon figurehead used to have glowing red eyes and a steam-spewing mouth; these days you'll have to content yourself with brightly colored shields and a red-and-white striped Viking sail with a big black eagle on it. At the next *really* high tide, the chain-saw-carved cowboys and Indians in the parking lot plan to climb aboard and sail to freedom.

The World-Famous Tree House: six miles south of Piercy, one-quarter mile south of Confusion Hill on the west side of Highway 101; clearly visible from the road. Open in summer, daily, 7 A.M.–8 P.M.; rest of the year, daily, 8 A.M.–5 P.M. Admission: free. Phone: (707) 925-6406.

The burnt-out interior of this gargantuan redwood is 50 feet high, making it—according to *Ripley's Believe It or Not!*—the tallest room in the world. A yellowish light bulb shines down from the unfathomable heights through decades' worth of cobwebs and dust. Antique coin-operated mechanical toys occupy the ground level. The trunk's rear exit leads, conveniently enough, into a gift shop.

POPE VALLEY
(Nine miles northeast of St. Helena)

Litto Damonte's Hubcap Ranch: From St. Helena, go northwest on Highway 29 for one mile and turn right (north) on Deer Park Road. Stay on Deer Park Road, which will become Howell Mountain Road, through Angwin north to Pope Valley. Turn left at the Pope Valley Garage, pass the Pope Valley Store and continue northwest on Pope Valley Road for two miles. The Hub cap Ranch is plainly visible on the right side of the road. Always visible. Admission: free.

Next time you pull over to the side of the road to pick up an interesting-looking hubcap, ponder what you might be getting yourself into. Litto Damonte did the same thing long ago, and ended up on a 30-year hubcap binge. He covered his ranch, fences, and driveway with hubcaps and more hubcaps. Then, to keep the hubcaps company, he started in on bird cages, tires, styrofoam surfboards, shells, cans, and reflectors. Damonte's family keeps the ranch just as Litto left it when he died. Passengers, take note: When the driver of the car you're riding in gets out to look around, pop off his hubcaps and hang them on the fence. Your driver will never be able to find his own among the thousands. Be prepared to walk home.

REDCREST
(22 miles north of Garberville)

Eternal Tree House: From Highway 101, take the Avenue of the Giants as it crosses to the east side of the highway just north of Founders Grove; the Avenue of the Giants goes through Redcrest, and the Eternal Tree House is on the northern edge of town, on the left (west) side of the road. Signs point the way. Open daily, daylight hours. Admission: free. Phone: (707) 722-4262.

The top of this once-giant tree was cut down early in this century; the remaining stump, as it turned out, had been hollowed out by fire and used by Indians and early settlers as a refuge. Now the 20-foot-high natural redwood room has moved on to a more glamorous lifestyle as a tourist attraction. Don't confuse this with the nearby Immortal Tree, which is just a plain ol' tree that never got chopped down.

REDDING

Lake Shasta Caverns: Take Highway 5 north from Redding 16 miles to the O'Brien/Shasta Caverns exit. Continue east on Shasta Caverns Road two miles to the Cavern Headquarters, where the road ends. Open April–October, daily, 9 A.M.–4 P.M., with tours every hour on the hour; November–March, daily, with tours at 10 A.M., noon, and 2 P.M. Admission: $9; children 4–12, $4; children under 4, free. Phone: (916) 238-2341.

This cave is so isolated that you'll quickly understand why it wasn't opened to the public until 1964. Visitors are ferried across the lake in catamarans and are loaded into buses and taken up to the caves, where they still have to do some walking to get inside. The extensive, pristine caves have many inappropriately named formations, such as Snow White and the Seven Dwarves, Garfield, the Spaghetti Patch, and Injun Charlie; but most are left, mercifully, to your imagination. We had fun looking at the bats. "Unfortunately, we do not have enough bats to capitalize on their droppings for fertilizer," laments the brochure. A pity.

ROHNERT PARK
(Seven miles south of Santa Rosa)

Gravity Anomaly: in the Sonoma Mountains. Exit Highway 101 east at Rohnert Park; drive east on Rohnert Park Expressway or East Cotati Avenue until you come to Petaluma Hill Road. Go south until you come to Roberts Road; turn left (east) on Roberts Road for one mile until you come to Lichau Road. Turn right on Lichau Road, which climbs steeply; after about three miles the road will take a sharp right turn, cross a cattle guard, and go into a dip. The anomaly is at the bottom of the dip. Always visible. Admission: free. For more information, call (707) 762-2785.

At the bottom of the dip on Lichau Road, turn off your car, put it in neutral, and watch what happens. Your car will roll *uphill* back toward the cattle guard. Get out and experiment with various round objects. They too will roll uphill. The standard explanation is, of course, "It's an optical illusion." Hmm. Nobody's done any scientific examination of this obscure mystery spot, so the verdict is still out. Watch out for other vehicles, as the local residents aren't too pleased with cars and bowling balls rolling uphill and blocking their road.

SANTA ROSA

Peanuts Museum and Gallery: 1667 West Steele Lane (at Cleveland), upstairs at the gift shop next to the Redwood Ice Arena, northwest end of the city. Open daily, 10 A.M.–6 P.M. Admission: free. Phone: (707) 546-7147.

Good grief! What's a Peanuts Gallery doing next to an ice rink in Santa Rosa? Well, Charles Schulz owns the place. The history of Charlie Brown et al. is traced from its beginnings—back when the humor in the strip was more like Family Circus. The characters really *have* aged over the years. Early strips, old sketches, original drawings, awards, and Peanuts-related artifacts are more than enough to awe any budding cartoonist or Schulz groupie.

Robert L. Ripley Memorial Museum: 492 Sonoma Avenue, on the north side of Julliard Park, just west of the intersection of Santa Rosa Avenue and Sonoma Avenue. Open May 16–August, Tuesday–Sunday, 11 A.M.–4 P.M.; September–Christmas, Wednesday–Sunday, 11 A.M.–4 P.M.; March–May 15, Wednesday–Sunday, 11 A.M.–4 P.M.; closed Christmas–February. Admission: $1; children 9–17, 50¢; seniors, 75¢; children under 9, free. Phone: (707) 576-5233.

This isn't a Ripley's Believe It or Not! museum but a museum about Ripley the person, and thus the only *real* Ripley museum in the world. Ripley, a Santa Rosa native, was one of the most popular cartoonists of all time. (The other most popular cartoonist, Charles Schulz, lives here, too. Has anybody ever checked the city's water supply?) Along with Ripley's personal effects—suitcases, clothing, original sketches—you'll see items from his curious collection: a two-headed, six-legged calf (calves?); a "real" fur-bearing trout; a flute made of a human bone. The museum itself is housed in an architectural oddity: a former church built from the wood of a single tree.

SEBASTOPOL

Pet-a-Llama Ranch: 5505 Lone Pine Road, off the Gravenstein Highway, south of town. Open Saturday–Sunday, 10 A.M.–4 P.M. Admission: free. Phone: (707) 823-9395.

The name Pet-a-Llama was the last word in cuteness, back when the ranch was located in the town of Petaluma. Now, however, the ranch must stand on its own merits. For free, you can pet the 17 llamas who live here; for 25¢ you can feed them. For more than that, you can take home a blanket made of their wool.

TULELAKE

(Four miles south of the Oregon border, near Klamath Falls)

Lava Beds National Monument: about 15 miles south of Tulelake. From Redding, turn east off Highway 5 onto Highway 299; continue east all the way to Canby, where you turn north on Highway 139. After 28 miles, there is a sign indicating a left (west) turn on Road 97, which goes through Tionesta to the Visitors' Center. The park is open and visible anytime; the Visitors' Center is open June 15–Labor Day, daily, 8 A.M.–6 P.M.; Labor Day–June 14, daily 8 A.M.–5 P.M. Admission: $3 per car when the Visitors' Center is open; free when it is closed. Phone: (916) 667-2282.

The first war we ever lost was Vietnam—right? Not exactly. The United States got its tail whupped in the little-known Modoc War of 1872–73. Eventually, the government did round up the pesky Modoc Indians, who were after all simply defending their own territory—but only after the Modocs (who had decimated and driven off the attacking soldiers) had left the battlefield, thinking the war was over. You can visit various battle sites, including Captain Jack's Stronghold, where the Modocs fended off an entire army that outnumbered them 20 to one. The rest of Lava Beds is a land of striking geological wonders: ice-coated lava tubes, freakish rock formations, cinder cones, and lava-glob "castles."

WEAVERVILLE

Joss House State Historic Park: corner of Oregon and Main Streets. Open in summer, daily, 10 A.M.–4:30 P.M.; tours depart every half-hour. In winter, open Thursday–Monday, 10 A.M.–4 P.M.; tours depart hourly. Admission: $1; children 6–17, 50¢; children under 6, free (but not recommended). Phone: (916) 623-5284.

Incense and offerings tell you that this is still a place of prayer. Chinese come from all over the country to see the temple, which was built around 1852 to serve Weaverville's Chinatown. It's more a blend of folk religions than a purely Taoist temple. Also on display here are weapons used in the Weaverville War, a gold-rush-era conflict between hostile Chinese tongs.

WILLOW CREEK
(35 miles east of Arcata)

Bigfoot Daze: Labor Day weekend. Parade begins at 10 A.M. and travels along Highway 299, through the center of town. For more information, call (707) 629-2693.

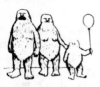

In Willow Creek, you might not see Bigfoot, stumble across one of his 16-inch footprints, or get a whiff of his knockout odor. But chances are, you'll meet someone who *has*. Hodgson's Store (Highway 299, west end of town) has plaster casts of Bigfoot footprints, and a map showing nearby places where people have spotted the shaggy 700-pounder in the past 30 years. At the Visitors' Center (corner of Highways 299 and 96), you can exchange squints with a 12-foot Bigfoot statue. At the Bigfoot Daze festival, enthusiasts come from all over the world to trade tales about the one that got away.

OREGON

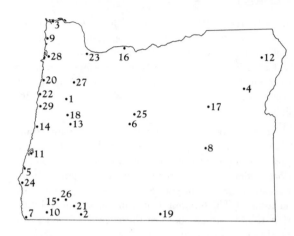

Legend:
1. Albany
2. Ashland
3. Astoria
4. Baker
5. Bandon
6. Bend
7. Brookings
8. Burns
9. Cannon Beach
10. Cave Junction
11. Coos Bay
12. Enterprise
13. Eugene
14. Florence
15. Grants Pass
16. Hood River
17. John Day
18. Junction City
19. Lakeview
20. Lincoln City
21. Medford
22. Newport
23. Portland
24. Port Orford
25. Redmond
26. Rogue River
27. Salem
28. Tillamook
29. Waldport

The rest of the country tends to forget that Oregon exists. They don't do it to be mean or anything. At least, we don't think so. Maybe it's just that the bigness of California elbows its quiet, forest-primeval neighbor aside, the way brash streetlights tend to erase the stars in the night sky.

And Oregon, for one reason or another, does not strive overly hard to make an impression on strangers. Things like Oregon blackberries and Tillamook cheese drift tantalizingly out of the state, but mostly Oregon goes about its own business, leaving others to scratch their heads and wonder about this cryptic land of woods, waves, and lava beds; of rooster-crowing contests, stilt races, and Duck Bingo.

Many of Oregon's weirdest attractions may not have been built with *you* in mind. But that makes them all the more worth investigating.

ALBANY

Slack Water Drift: last Sunday in July. Official starting point is behind Michael's Landing restaurant off the highway on the Willamette River, at 603 Northwest 2nd in Corvallis, at 9 A.M. The "drift" continues down the river until it reaches Albany. You can join in at any point. For more information, call KGAL at (503) 926-8683.

The theme of this anti-race is to be lazy, waste time, squirt your neighbors with water pistols, and float aimlessly down the river. If you're ambitious, you can build a floating dragon, "drive" the hull of a car strapped to plastic barrels, or dine in your Sunday finest on board your aqua-bistro. The funniest floats win prizes from radio station KGAL, which sponsors the event. All you really need to join are an inner tube, a swimming suit, and the spirit of summer.

ASHLAND

Backstage Tour: purchase tickets at the Box Office, off Main Street at the entrance to Lithia Park. Tours depart from the Black Swan Theatre during Oregon Shakespeare Festival season, every performance day at 10 A.M. Admission: $6; children, $3. Phone: (503) 482-4331. Advance reservations are recommended.

The two-hour tour, often guided by a genuine actor or stagehand, lets you prowl backstage areas; dressing rooms; a costuming shop; and the "touchy-feely room," in which you can handle props actually used in the Ashland plays, such as swords and fake body parts. A tour highlight is a visit to the Exhibit Center (which you can visit separately for $1; children, 50¢), a sort of Shakespeare Festival museum with changing displays of costumes, props, and photos relating to current shows.

Continuum Exhibit: 1813 Highway 99 North, in the Bear Valley Commercial Center Mall; take bus 10 north from downtown Ashland. Open Monday–Saturday, 10 A.M.–5 P.M.; Sunday, 11 A.M.–5 P.M. Admission: $2; students, $1; children under 10 free with adult. Phone: (503) 488-1032.

You're smug now. But one day, sucker, you gonna die! Then what? Your body will be at the bottom of the East River, and your soul...where will your soul be? The Continuum Exhibit tackles that big question, though it doesn't come up with any dogmatic answers. You're supposed to think about your own answers. The maze of slick display boards concentrates on one possibility: life after death. Learn about Kirlian photography; quantum physics; multicultural conceptions of the afterlife; cryogenics; the insubstantiality of matter; and what Plato, Einstein, and Mother Teresa had to say on the subject. A creepy hologram shows how stupid you're gonna feel after you commit suicide.

Shakespeare Art Museum: 460 B Street, two blocks north of Main Street. Open April–October, Wednesday–Sunday, 10 A.M.–5 P.M. Also, summer Monday-night "open houses," 7–9 P.M. Admission: $2; open houses are free. Phone: (503) 488-0332.

Behind this prim title is one radical art museum: an artistic id hooked on the Bard and holding a perceptive funhouse mirror up to his plays. Hannah Tompkins has spent 56 years studying Shakespeare. Her impressionistic works reveal weird, hidden aspects of the plays and the human relationships therein. "Merchant of Venice" depicts a Christlike figure and a skull peering out of a box. Don't miss Tompkins' Shakespearean Tarot Deck, in which the suits are represented by the Evil-Doers, the Status-Seekers, the Fated Ones, and the Fools.

ASTORIA

Scandinavian Midsummer Festival: the weekend nearest June 21, Friday–Sunday. All events except parade are held at Astoria High School on West Marine Drive, just off Highway 202. Admission: $2.50; children 5–12, $1; children under 5, free. Phone: (503) 325-6311.

People in costume erect a flower-bedecked midsummer pole and dance around it, not once mentioning the pointed symbolism of such an act. Another festival highlight is a hex-burning bonfire to destroy evil spirits. A rough-and-tumble tug-of-war pits various Scandinavian ethnicities against each other; accordion concerts, craft booths, and Scandinavian meals round out the festival.

BAKER

Gold Nugget Display: in the U.S. National Bank of Oregon's lobby, 2000 Main Street (at Washington). Open Monday–Thursday, 10 A.M.–5 P.M.; Friday, 10 A.M.–6 P.M. Admission: free. Phone: (503) 523-7791.

There's gold in them thar glass cases! The star of this show is the whopping seven-pound Armstrong Nugget. Plenty of other oddly shaped, mouth-watering nuggets share the shelves with old gold coins and gold dust and gold flakes and gold, gold, gold! We're headin' west, Nettie—I've got the fever!

Porcupine and Rubber Duck Races: at the Miners' Jubilee, third weekend in July. Rubber duck race: Saturday, 3 P.M., starting at Broadway Street Bridge. Porcupine races: Saturday, 7:30 P.M., Baker High School stadium, 2500 E Street. Bed races: Sunday, noon, Grove Street between Campbell and Madison Streets. For more information, call (503) 523-5855.

Prospectors of yore would spin in their graves if they knew what Baker is doing in the name of miners. The local 4-H club catches porcupines ("porkies," they call 'em around here) in the woods and rents them to people who want to race the critters. You're also allowed to bring your own porcupine to the race. All participants are strictly forbidden to poke their porcupines with brooms. (That's in the rules.) The rubber duck race is a less prickly event, in which all ducks are given code numbers and dumped in the Powder River. They're retrieved downriver; the fastest ducks entitle their owners to prizes. A madcap bed race is Sunday's big event. After the Jubilee, the porcupines are returned to their natural habitat, as are the rubber ducks and the beds.

BANDON

Sand Castle/Sand Sculpture Contest: Memorial Day. On the beach, off Beach Loop Drive at Seabird Lane. Construction begins at 9 A.M.; judging is at 1 P.M. For more information, call (503) 347-9616.

Here in the self-declared Storm Capital of the World, competitors get pretty serious, as there are several hundred dollars at stake. Giant animals, nautical fantasy scenes, and famous people's profiles are all earnestly sculpted, and just as earnestly gobbled up by King Neptune at the end of the day.

BEND

Lava Cast Forest: 14 miles south of town on Highway 97; go past the Lava River Cave turnoff and turn left (east) on Forest Road 9720 (across from the Sunriver turnoff) and stay on that road for nine miles until it ends. Open when weather permits. Admission: free. Phone: (503) 593-2421.

Ancient lava flows swallowed up trees throughout this area; a layer of lava hardened around the noncharred trees as the lava flow level lowered. Eventually, over the centuries, the burnt trees rotted away and the casts around them became hollow. The result today is an arboreal Herculaneum: an antiforest, acknowledged as the world's largest. Most of the lava cast stumps are only a few feet above the new ground level, but the holes go down 10 to 20 feet to the old ground level. Antilogs, looking like stone-age water pipes, dot the landscape.

Lavacicle Cave: 45 miles southeast of Bend. Tours leave from the Pine Mountain Ranger Station. To make a reservation (and get directions to the station), call the Lava Lands Visitors' Center at (503) 593-2421. Tours are given May–September, third Saturday of every month, 8:30 A.M.–1:30 P.M. Admission: free.

Are you prepared to *crawl* into the bowels of the earth? After 50 feet of crawling, you've got to squat for another 50 feet. After that, it's clear sailing all the way. The question on your lips now might be, "Why would I want to see a lavacicle if you won't even tell me what it is?" Good point. Lavacicles are stalactites and stalagmites created not by the slow dripping accumulation of minerals but by semimolten lava oozing off the ceiling of a newly formed cave. And this cave's got lots of 'em. The isolation, darkness, and strange formations make this a top-notch—if somewhat top-secret—subterranean experience.

Lava River Cave: 12 miles south of Bend, off Highway 97; keep going past the Oregon High Desert Museum and turn left (east) at the sign for the Lava River Cave Office. Open mid-May–mid-September, daily, 9 A.M.–6 P.M. Admission: $1; students 12–17, 50¢; children under 12, free. Phone: (503) 593-2421.

This is just about the best example anywhere of that rare volcanic creature, the lava tube. Bring a flashlight (or rent one at the entrance, 50¢), because there's no lighting for us human intruders. The cave was formed when the outer sides of a lava flow hardened; the interior, still molten, flowed away, leaving a mile-long tube that was eventually covered up by erosion of nearby hills. Don't expect funny names and punning tour guides. This is a serious cave. Keep an eye out for lavacicles and intriguing sand formations, an ear out for distorted echoes, and your ESP sensors out for things that go bump in the dark.

BLITZEN
(80 miles south of Burns)

Ghost Town: Go south from Burns on Highway 205 until you reach Frenchglen; continue south 15 more miles until you reach Roaring Springs Ranch (not marked on all maps). Highway 205 officially ends here but the road continues. Keep going south on what is now a gravel road for about three miles until you come to a dirt road branching right (west); follow this dirt road west, keeping to the left (south) when you come to a branch in the road. After about three miles this road will run through the center of Blitzen. Access is free and unrestricted. For more information in case you get lost, try the Burns Historical Society at (503) 573-2163 or the Frenchglen Hotel at (503) 493-2825.

Don't look for Blitzen on the map. Don't even look for the roads that lead to Blitzen on the map. Blitzen is about as obscure a ghost town as you'll ever find (or not find), having eluded the notice of even the most ardent ghost-town hunters. Yet there it stands—barely: about six buildings struggling to stay upright. It was a ranching town, not a mining town, so don't expect to find buried gold or ore tracings. The old schoolhouse (later used as a speakeasy) braves the winds, as do a garage, a barn, a store, a house, and some shacks. Ruins and foundations add to the ghostly air. This is technically on private property, so taking or vandalizing anything is strictly verboten.

BROOKINGS

Beachcombers' Festival: usually the third weekend in March (dates depend on spring break; call to confirm). Saturday, 9 A.M.–7 P.M.; Sunday, 9 A.M.–4 P.M. Held at Azalea Middle School, 505 Pacific Street (at Oak). Admission: $1.50; students, 50¢. One admission ticket is good for both days. For more information, call (503) 469-4929 or (503) 469-3181.

Remember that great piece of driftwood you once found? The one that looked exactly like Grace Kelly in a fuzzy robe? You'll see even better ones at Brookings' annual driftwood show, where hundreds of devoted beachcombers exhibit art made from the fruits of their combing: collages; mobiles; driftwood in funny shapes; driftwood made into useful objects; driftwood waxed and unwaxed, decorated and undecorated. Throughout the weekend, a program of slide shows, films, and lectures celebrates beach culture.

BROWNSVILLE
(25 miles northeast of Eugene)

The Living Rock Studios: 911 Bishop Way West. Open Tuesday–Saturday, 10 A.M.–5 P.M.; Sunday, 2–6 P.M. Admission: donation. Phone: (503) 466-5814.

To make his "studios" of "living rock," the more-than-eccentric Howard Taylor carefully glued together multicolored translucent semiprecious stones, forming intricate Bible scenes. Then he backlit them with fluorescent bulbs. You haven't truly experienced life until you've seen a glowing rhodonite Moses or a Burning Bush made of opalized carnelian.

BURNS

Bed Race: last Saturday in June. Costume contest: 9 A.M., Elks Club parking lot, Madison and Broadway. Bed parade: 9:30 A.M., down Broadway. Bed race: 10 A.M., also down Broadway. For more information, call (503) 573-2934.

Participants dress in authentic nightwear, and each bed is "dressed" according to the local business that sponsors it. Thus you can imagine what the Burns Nursing Home's bed might look like, and the local Safeway store's. Comedy is all well and good, but speed is the key factor as each bed makes several fast trips down Broadway.

Malheur Cave: Go southwest from Burns on Highway 78, past New Princeton, to a cinder dirt road turnoff on the left (northeast) side of the road; take this three miles to the cave. The cave is owned by the Burns Masonic Lodge and is open only by special arrangement, anytime except during August, when they have their meetings in the cave. To arrange for a permission slip and a key to the gate, call one of the Masonic officers: Alan Basey at (503)

573-2757, Gene Mackey at (503) 573-7458, Lee Wallace at (503) 573-2679 or, as a last resort, the Masonic Lodge at (503) 573-2220. There are two gates on the road to the cave; the second one is locked; thus the key.

Five hundred feet into the cave you'll come to the bleachers that the Masons installed for their secret meetings. Beyond these is a rock and mud pile, which makes the going a little rough, especially considering the total darkness and the ghosts of Indians and Masons flitting about. After a while you'll come to—surprise!—the shores of an underground lake, which stretches off into the inky blackness. From here on in you need a boat; sometimes you'll find one tied up on the shore. Once out on the water, look above for "lava straws" and look below for sunken boats on the bottom of the lake. The water continues all the way to the end of the winding cave, where a secret cache of gems and gold nuggets awaits you. Oops—was that supposed to be a secret?

CANNON BEACH

Sand Castle Contest: the lowest-tide Saturday in late May (varies, depending on the tides). On the beach, one-quarter mile north of Haystack Rock. Building begins in early morning; judging starts around noon. For more information, call (503) 436-2623.

Oregon's most prestigious sand castle contest is also the state's original one, dreamed up 25 years ago by three women who were determined to put Cannon Beach on the map. Over 1,000 contestants show up armed with shovels, squirt bottles, and surprisingly complicated plans. Recent winners included a whale-sized sea turtle, the pyramids of Egypt, and a lifelike tugboat.

CAVE JUNCTION
(28 miles southwest of Grants Pass)

Middle Earth: 24553 Redwood Highway (Highway 199), two miles north of Cave Junction in the town of Kerby, on the east side of the road. Open daily, 9 A.M.–dusk, weather permitting. Admission: free. Phone: (503) 592-4445.

This place makes the locals edgy. "It's got a funny sign with a demon jumping around on it," says one. But the owner shrugs it off, insisting that he put some painted plywood Hobbit-shaped cutouts out by the highway simply to entice tourists to stop at his gift shop. Along with the litany of Tolkein characters, take note of the Hobbit House, a tiny photogenic shack; a waterfall with a little castle on top; and a picnic ground that shares the Middle Earth theme. The gift shop sells fantasy figurines; Tolkein and occultism books; and other things related to unicorns, fairies, and other legendary creatures. Goofy gift shop or Demonology World Headquarters? You decide.

Oregon Caves: 20 miles east of town at the end of Highway 46 (Caves Highway). Open June 10–September 11, daily, 8 A.M.–7 P.M.; May 1–June 9 and September 12–September 30, daily, 9 A.M.–5 P.M.; October 1–April 30, daily, 10:30 A.M.–12:30 P.M. and 2–3:30 P.M. Admission: $5.75; children 6–11, $3; children under 6 not admitted, but there is a $3 baby-sitting service. Phone: (503) 592-3400.

Where in Oregon can you find the Banana Grove, Neptune's Grotto, Niagara Falls, the Passageway of the Whale, and the Ghost Room? Underground, here at the Oregon Caves. The names belong to stalagmites, stalactites and oozing stone formations. When they can't figure out what a particular formation looks like, they dub it "The Imagination Room." We think every room should be called "The Imagination Room," as cave formations are really nature's three-dimensional Rorschach test. Giving names to oddly shaped stalactites is like saying to your subject, "Here's an inkblot shaped like a pelvic bone. What do you think it looks like?" This is a chilly cave—41 degrees year-round—so bring your earmuffs.

Trees of Wonder and Tractor Collection: on the grounds of the Fordson Home Hostel, 250 Robinson Road, near the town of Holland. From Cave Junction, go six miles east on Highway 46 (Caves Highway); turn right (south) on Holland Loop Road (at the Siskiyou Winery); this road will turn left, after which you should keep going straight, even though Holland Loop Road branches to the right. By going straight you will come to Robinson Road and the hostel. Open anytime, but the trees and tractors are only visible during daylight hours. Admission: Looking around the grounds is free; staying overnight at the hostel costs money. Call ahead to tell them you're coming. Phone: (503) 592-3203.

Tired of touristy Mystery Spots, yet looking for the Real Thing? Here it is. No admission fee; no accursed Mystery Shack. The people at the hostel will direct you to the 60-

by-200-foot area where the trees look like they're doing the shimmy, all curving inexplicably in one direction and then the other, and often growing as much as six degrees off from the vertical. Other plants shun the area, though they grow abundantly in the surrounding forest. Government and freelance scientists and botanists have studied the area, but to no avail. They usually end up more confused than when they started. Nearby is the owner's antique Fordson Tractor collection: over 15 creaking rarities that were once the Model T of the tractor world. The owner also has a collection of antique tractor *toys* inside the hostel. What's more, Bigfoot has recently been sighted in the immediate vicinity—even by people staying at the hostel.

COOS BAY

Seaman's Center: 171 North Broadway, center of town. Open evenings after 6 P.M. when ships are in port. Admission: free.

"Lemme tell you 'bout the time, off the coast of Sumatra, how I got this here wooden leg," says old Cap'n Mickles, clutching his glass. Your eyes drift to the exotica perched on dusty shelves as Mickles spins his dubious yarn of harpoons and Indonesian pirates. On display are coins and bills from every country that has even an inch of coastline. Model ships made by retired sailors compete for space with baskets, banners, and oriental curios, souvenirs of long-gone voyages. Most of Coos Bay's lumber shipping trade is with the Orient, so this funky café/club, where the sailing men while away their evenings while waiting to ship out, is a repository for tall tales and mysterious knickknacks bought in the back alleys of Singapore. Try to look worldly and weatherbeaten if you don't want to stick out like a sore thumb.

CORNUCOPIA
(64 miles northeast of Baker)

Ghost Town: 12 miles northeast of Halfway on a paved road that becomes a gravel road after five miles. Halfway is 52 miles east of Baker on Highway 86.

This ghost town has about four buildings standing, but you know how it is with ghost towns: "Standing" has a broad definition. Many parts of the old mining buildings huddle weak-kneed in the wind; several other structures of undetermined function have totally succumbed to gravity. A few miners occasionally occupy trailers nearby.

FLORENCE

The American Museum of Fly Fishing: 280 Nopal Street, three blocks north of the Old Town waterfront. Open daily, 10 A.M.–5 P.M. Admission: $2.50; children under 16, free. Phone: (503) 997-6102.

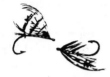

What's weirder than a fish out of water? A fishing fly captured in a frame. You'll see thousands of them here, seductive twists of hair and feathers lashed to fishhooks of all sizes, meticulously mounted and framed by master framer William Cushner. Alongside the flies in each frame are fishy paintings and wooden fish so lifelike that visitors have asked Cushner who taxidermed them. Note the tiny flies attached to quarter-inch hooks. Weirdest of all is that Cushner himself neither fishes nor ties flies. "What's the point?" he says.

Indian Forest: 88493 Highway 101 North, four miles north of town on the east side of the highway. Look for the totem pole out front. Open June–August, daily, 8 A.M.–dusk; May, September, and October, daily, 10 A.M.–4 P.M. Closed November–April. Admission: $3; children 12–18, $2; children 5–11, $1.50; children under 5, free. Phone: (503) 997-3677.

A wooded path winds past life-size replicas of Native American dwellings. Birds twitter in the bush, deepening your sense of meandering undisturbed through Indian encampments as you enter and explore the Navajo hogan, Ojibwa wigwam, Sioux tipi, an underground lodge, and more. An Oregon structural engineer built the dwellings 20 years ago after careful research; his love of buildings got him started on the project. Also notable here are the life-size plastic horse blandly guarding the tipi, and a herd of real buffalo, who scowl darkly into your camera.

National Stilt Walking Championship: July 4, 2 P.M. Starts at the corner of Maple and Bay Streets in Old Town. Anyone can enter. Registration (no charge) starts at 1 P.M. Use the stilts provided or bring your own. For more information, call (503) 997-2963 or (503) 997-3128.

It's not how fast you can go that matters; it's how long you can stay up and how far you can go. The stilts are the long kind that you steady with your hands; foot stirrups are one to two feet off the ground. The course goes up and down downtown streets, which are closed to traffic for the event. The 1988 champion managed nearly three miles. You can top that. Easy.

Sea Lion Caves: on the west side of Highway 101, 11 miles north of Florence. Enter through the gift shop. Open daily, 9 A.M.–one hour before dark (usually 7 P.M. in summer, 4:30 P.M. in winter). Jackets and binoculars are recommended year-round. Admission: $4; children 6–15, $2.50; children under 6, free. Phone: (503) 547-3111.

In fall and winter, a herd of wild Steller sea lions whoops it up inside the cavern, which is America's largest sea cave, 12 stories high and covering two acres, striated with mineral hues. In spring and summer the sea lions dwell outside the cave on adjacent rocky ledges, where you can watch the deep-throated bulls putting on their macho act.

Slug Race: third Saturday in May. Bay Street at Nopal, on the Old Town waterfront. Phone: (503) 997-3128.

This race is part of Florence's Rhododendron Festival, the West Coast's second oldest festival. But you don't care about rhododendrons; you care about gastropods. Members of the local variety, a modest three inches long, are placed in a circle and encouraged to come out. Take this opportunity to buy a local specialty: a slug recipe cookbook. It's strictly tongue-in-cheek, say the Florentines, and not slug-in-cheek. It's for sale at Old Town gift shops.

FOREST GROVE
(25 miles west of Portland)

Barbershop Ballad and Beard-Growing Contest: usually the first weekend in March. Pacific University Field House, North Main Street, north-central part of town. Competitions and shows start at 6:10 P.M., Friday and Saturday. Tickets (various prices) available in advance and at the door. For more information, call (503) 357-6006.

There's something perverse about having a *barbershop* ballad contest and a *beard*-growing contest at the same time. Guess they're trying to be an equal-opportunity city. Your whole body will resonate when you listen to these very serious balladeers. A series of elimination bouts on Friday set the stage for the knock-down drag-out croon-a-thon Saturday evening. The beard event is part of a Gay '90s parade on Saturday. From 10 A.M.–noon on Main Street, judges award prizes to the owners of the longest, neatest, bushiest, sexiest, and "kissiest" beards in town.

GARIBALDI
(Ten miles north of Tillamook)

Crab Races: a weekend in February (varies). Starts at 9 A.M., at the Ghost Hole Tavern, Highway 101 (at 4th). Crab Rental: $1. Race is in the tavern's parking lot; minors are not allowed inside the tavern. For current date and more information, call (503) 322-0215 or (503)322-0301.

Generations of Garibaldians have made their living hauling Dungeness crabs out of the sea. Finally somebody got the idea to humiliate the crabs before cooking them. A four-by-eight-foot sheet is marked with lanes, and the crabs—never fond of walking in a straight line—scuttle confusedly about. Winners compete in the big Crescent City (California) crab races.

GOLD HILL
(12 miles northwest of Medford)

The Oregon Vortex House of Mystery: 4303 Sardine Creek Road. Exit from Highway 5 to Highway 234 through Gold Hill to Sardine Creek Road, just one mile north of Gold Hill. Turn east on Sardine Creek Road for four miles. Open June–August, daily, 9 A.M.–4:45 P.M.; March–May and September–October 15, Friday–Tuesday, 9 A.M.–4:45 P.M.; closed October 16–February. Admission: $3.50; children 12–15, $2.50; children 5–11, $1.50; children under 5, free. Phone: (503) 855-1543.

This, the undisputed patriarch of Mystery Spots, has had a long history of ups and downs. When that cabin slid down the hill to become the world's first Mystery Shack, that was no tragedy. That was good for business. In 1987, *Omni* magazine ran an article that "proved" that the vortex was only a clever optical illusion. Luckily, most people who visit the vortex do not read *Omni*. So the Oregon Vortex strides onward, officiously dismissing all other Mystery Spots as pathetic imitators. And the truth is, they *are* imitators, since (as far as anyone can tell) this was the very first one to charge admission. Having imitators, though, doesn't mean you were authentic in the first place.

GRANTS PASS

Caveman Mascot: corner of NE Morgan Lane and NE 6th Street, in the small triangular park near the Shell station, at the north end of town next to Highway 5.

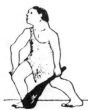

In 1922, a group of visionaries decided that Josephine County, home of the Oregon Caves, needed a mascot. What else but a caveman? Never mind that the Oregon Caves never housed cavemen. They dubbed their creation Joco the Friendly Caveman (Joco for JOsephine COunty). Now a towering, lumbering, 30-foot-tall colossus guards the entrance to Grants Pass, his dim eyes scanning the horizon. If you attend a local festival, don't be alarmed at the arrival of a band of wild Neanderthals wreaking havoc in full animal-skin regalia. They're the Oregon Cavemen, the "world's most unique booster group."

Renaissance Fair: the weekend closest to the middle of July. Riverside Park, south of downtown, next to the Rogue River. Festival runs Saturday, 9 A.M.–9 P.M.; Sunday, 9 A.M.–6 P.M. For current dates and other information, call (503) 474-7459.

There's no *e* on the end of the title of this event, and we just don't know how they can do without it. The 16th-century atmosphere is enhanced by wandering minstrels, jousting knights, jugglers, and Shakespearean actors. Velvet-clad hopefuls (you, perhaps?) compete for prizes in the Kings and Paupers costume parade. Nearly 100 booths offer Renaissance-type crafts and food, or close enough to it for horseshoes.

HILLSBORO
(18 miles west of Portland)

Storybook Rockery: in the yard of an unnumbered white house on Farmington Road, two doors down from the

Twin Oaks Tavern. Open April–October, daily, daylight hours. Admission: discretionary donation. Phone: (503) 628-1575.

What began as a penchant for making gingerbread houses has grown, since 1966, into a rocky wonderland. One lady built all 65 of the little rock and cement storybook houses here. Measuring from one to five-and-a-half feet tall, each house is completely different from the others—glass windows here, a chubby chimney there. The houses are peopled with ceramic characters: Jack Horner, Miss Muffet, and their ilk. It'll make you darn sorry you ever grew up.

HOOD RIVER
(60 miles east of Portland)

Luhr Jensen Fishing Lure Company: 400 Portway Street, on the riverfront. Half-hour tours are given Tuesday and Thursday, 11 A.M. and 1:30 P.M. Admission: free. Phone: (503) 386-3811.

Vast numbers of burly, wool-hat-wearing men and women think hooking fish is just as fun as heck. Here at one of Oregon's biggest plastic and metal lure manufacturers, you can witness firsthand the brightly colored ingenuity that goes into tricking those elusive Professor Moriartys of the deep.

St. Urho's Day: March 16. Parade begins at 10 A.M. and travels down Oak Street. For more information, call (503) 386-1802 or (503) 386-2000.

St. Urho—slayer of grasshoppers, and Finland's answer to St. Patrick—once encountered a horde of locusts bent on devouring Finland's entire wine-grape crop. Urho chanted gravely, in Finnish, "Grasshopper, grasshopper, go to hell." So they did. Hood River's wry parade features locals dressed as locusts. The Urhomobile, a VW bug in lime green and purple (green for the bugs, purple for the grapes) rumbles down the street as everybody chants, "Grasshopper, grasshopper, go to hell" (in Finnish, yet). After the parade, everyone retires to their favorite bar and drinks—what else?—grasshoppers. A Finnish potluck dinner at the Crag Rat Hut is followed by a tall-tale contest. All tales must be about St. Urho and be told in "Finnglish."

JACKSONVILLE
(Five miles west of Medford)

Beekman House Historical Re-enactment: 452 East California Street (at Laurelwood). Open Memorial Day–Labor Day, daily, 1–5 P.M. Admission: free, but donations are welcomed. Phone: (503) 899-1847.

Outside the Beekman House, it's 1989. Inside, it's 1911: furniture, newspapers, clothing, attitudes—everything. The actors playing wealthy banker C. C. Beekman, his family, and his servants show you around their house, speaking of "current" events and treating you like a family friend. Various 1911 characters—maids, repairmen, students—wander in and out, and no one misses a beat. As you emerge into the light of the present day, the sensation can only be described as disoriented melancholy.

JEFFERSON
(Ten miles northeast of Albany)

Frog Jumping Championship: third Sunday in July. Downtown, in the bank parking lot on Main Street. Races begin at 1 P.M., end at 5 P.M. For more information, call (503) 327-2241.

This is Oregon's only frog-jumping event. The only one. Bring your own frog or rent one for free on the day of the race. Heed the Jeffersonians' words of wisdom: A big frog is a muscular frog; but a too-big frog is too heavy to get off the ground.

JOHN DAY

Kam Wah Chung and Company Museum: 250 Northwest Canton, next to the city park in the Kam Wah Chung Historical Wayside. Open May–October, Monday–Thursday, 9 A.M.–noon and 1–5 P.M.; Saturday and Sunday, 1–5 P.M. Closed Friday. Admission: free, but donations are welcomed. Phone: (503) 575-0028.

In the 1880s, John Day had twice as many Chinese residents as caucasian ones. The building that houses this museum served, between the 1880s and the 1940s, as general store, herbal pharmacy, hotel, fortune-teller's studio, casino, assay office, and Taoist shrine. Today you can see traces of all these incarnations. On display are the herb doctor's personal effects, as well as herbs, packaged food, cigarettes, utensils, tea, and several shrines.

Mid-September finds the town celebrating Kam Wah Chung Days, complete with rickshaws and a dragon parade.

JOSEPH
(Seven miles south of Enterprise)

Wallowa Lake Monster Observation and Preservation Society Gala: third weekend in August. At the south end of Wallowa Lake, five miles south of Joseph, at the picnic grounds and marina. For more information, call (503) 426-4074.

Nessie gets all the publicity, but Wally—Wallowa Lake's very own monster—is a lot more fun. He's a real party monster. He hasn't been sighted since 1983, but that doesn't stop M.O.P.S. (the Monster Observation and Preservation Society) from hoping. The festivities begin Saturday morning and include a stage play about Wally and the offering of a sacrificial virgin (should the monster happen to show up hungry). At the "Submarine Race," a lady in a wetsuit peers into the water and gives a blow-by-blow narration. Of course, nobody can see the submarines. That's because they aren't there. The Society Picnic, on Sunday, features Monsterburgers.

JUNCTION CITY
(12 miles northwest of Eugene)

Scandinavian Festival: second weekend in August (usually Friday–Monday). Most activities take place on Greenwood Street, between 5th and 7th. Phone: (503) 998-6154 or (503) 998-3300.

Junction City, founded by Danish immigrants, is quick to point out that although the town is 5,433 miles from Sweden, it's a cozy 5,100 from beautiful downtown Denmark. For nearly 30 years the locals have celebrated their Norse roots with folk dance, food, crafts booths, and—best of all—playlets enacting Hans Christian Andersen's stories.

LAKEVIEW

The Fantastic Museum: two miles north of Lakeview on the west side of Highway 395, at Hunter's Hot Springs Resort. You can't miss it. Open Saturday and Sunday, 10 A.M.–8 P.M. If you ask nicely, they might let you in at other times, too. Admission: free, but donations are welcomed. Phone: (503) 947-2127.

Most of the stuff in here was on exhibit at the 1962 Seattle World's Fair. In storage for 20 years, it has finally been unearthed, moved to Lakeview, and combined with its new owners' own collection of odd knickknacks. A focal point here is Olaf, the mummified giant, a former sideshow freak. As legend has it, Olaf was stretched to death on a rack and then tossed into a Norwegian bog 650 years ago. The museum is full of talking mechanical automata that were cheesy antiques even back in 1962. And have you spent long hours wondering whatever became of Elvis' first guitar? Here it is. Added bonus: a collection of antique outhouses stands in a nearby field.

Old Perpetual Geyser: two miles north of Lakeview on the west side of Highway 395 at Hunter's Hot Springs Resort. Always open. Admission: free. Phone: (503) 947-2127.

Now that Old Faithful is surrounded by a million acres of wasteland, its overlooked Oregon cousin, Old Perpetual, should get some recognition at last. Old Perpetual spritzes 60 feet skyward every 90 seconds, giving the ducks around the geyser's pool a hot shower 960 times a day. Clean ducks. As far as we can tell, this is one of only three regularly spouting geysers in the whole country. (Calistoga [California] and Yellowstone have the others.)

LEBANON
(14 miles southeast of Albany)

Strawberry Festival: first full weekend in June (Friday–Sunday). In past years, festivities took place at the corner of 5th and Rose Streets, but the festival will move to a new location in 1989. For new location and other information, call (503) 258-7164.

Cut up and dished out for free on Saturday afternoon is the world's largest strawberry shortcake. (Check the *Guinness Book of World's Records* if you don't believe us.) Looming moistly on its huge platform, the oven-fresh behemoth stands much, much taller than you or I. Its weight is measured in terms of tonnage. Fresh strawberries are spooned over every slice.

LINCOLN CITY

Grass Carp Festival: second weekend in September. Activities take place at the Regatta Grounds on the west side of Devils Lake. Saturday–Sunday, 9 A.M.–6 P.M. Carp Festival Kit (windsock, T-shirt, pin): $15. For more information, call (503) 994-3070 or, in Oregon, (800) 452-2151.

When 700-acre Devils Lake became so weedbound as to render motorboating impossible, the city got mad as hell. They brought in 27,090 hungry grass carp from Arkansas and dumped 'em in the lake. The fish were all sterile; so, having nothing better to do, they ate. They cleared up the weed problem in a trice, and gained an alarming amount of weight. Now Lincoln City honors its huge scaly saviors with this festival. People cavort in wide-mouthed carp costumes; they fly grass carp windsocks and join the chorus of the official festival song, "You Gotta Have Carp."

Kite Festivals: The spring festival is Mothers' Day weekend; the fall festival is the last weekend in September. Activities take place at the D River Wayside, just off Highway 101. Exact time depends on the wind. For more information, call (503) 994-3070 or, in Oregon, (800) 452-2151.

Here in the self-declared Kite Capital of the World, home of kite limbo contests and whistling kites, you can marvel at the world's largest windsock: over 100 feet long and capable of carrying passengers. At night, people fly intensely glowing, weirdly colored night-kites. Prizes are awarded to the festival's most unusual kite, the best tiny (under eight inches) kite, the funniest kite, and the most innovative kite tail.

Mudflat Classic Golf Tournament: the lowest-tide Sunday in August. Siletz Bay Beach. Exact time depends on the tide. For current date and time, call (503) 994-3070, or in Oregon, (800) 452-2151.

When the tide goes out around here, it goes way, way out. The resultant mudflat becomes Oregon's stickiest golf course. Competitors use branches, plastic flamingoes, brooms, *anything* (even golf clubs) to whack golf balls into frisbeelike containers stuck in the ooze. The Mudflat Classic's incongruous companion event is a Daisy Mae look-alike contest. In recent years, to everyone's surprise, *men* have been sashaying away with the prizes.

Sand Castle Contest: the lowest-tide Saturday in August. Taft Dock, at Southwest 51st Street on Siletz Bay. For current date and more information, call (503) 994-3070, or in Oregon, (800) 452-2151.

Excitement and tension are so thick at this festival that you could slice them with a sand shovel. The reason? Competitors must complete their creations in a scant, hair-tearing 90-minute period. Craft booths line the sidewalk nearby, proffering arts and crafts.

Treasure Hunt: held throughout the seven days of spring break (dates are determined by the Oregon school system). Siletz Bay Beach. Phone: (503) 994-3070, or in Oregon, (800) 452-2151.

That's *buried* treasure, maties. Every morning for a week, festival officials sneak out to the beach in the wee, wee hours and bury real booty in the sand: $1,000 worth, in all. And all *you* need to do is wander up and down the strand all day searching for it. Among the buried goodies are silver coins and tokens and plastic-wrapped gift certificates for local stores. Hint: Many of the treasures are hidden among the logs and driftwood.

MARION
(13 miles northeast of Albany)

Llamaland: 14607 Duckflat Road Southeast. Open first and third Sundays of every month, noon–5 P.M. Admission: free. Phone: (503) 769-7297.

It's a wavy, woolly sea of llamas—200 in all, including a constant crop of cuddly new babies. This is a llama research center and not a ranch, so on the guided tour you'll learn about wool genetics, reproduction, and the whole zoological shebang. You can feed and pet the more spoiled and gregarious of the llamas.

NEHALEM
(22 miles north of Tillamook)

Duck Days: Presidents' Saturday (February). Events take place all over town, but the town is only two blocks long. SusQuack arrives by boat, 10 A.M., at the boat dock just off the Roy Harwood Square next to the Sanitary Authority. For more information, call (503) 368-6924.

Picture a big board with numbers printed all over it, and across the top, the letters B-I-N-G-O. Picture live ducks waddling excitedly all over the board, leaving squiggly deposits in their wake. And every time a duckdoo lands on a number, some happy gambler squeals with joy. That's no nightmare, that's Duck Bingo, a staple event at this festival. Also on the agenda are the waddle race; the eat-crackers-and-whistle contest; a rock-skipping contest (new special category for grandmothers); the big foot/small foot contest; and a look-alike contest in which competitors emulate SusQuack, the gigantic, hairy duck who is the festival's mascot.

NEWPORT

Ripley's Believe It or Not!: Mariner Square, 250 Southwest Bay Boulevard, next to the Waxworks. Open in summer, daily, 9 A.M.–8 P.M.; other times, daily, 10 A.M.–5 P.M. Admission: $4; students 12–17, $3; children 5–11, $2; children under 5, free. Phone: (503) 265-2206.

Another in the series of off-the-wall Ripley museums. Though they might look the same on the outside, they're all different inside. Highlights here include a dagger made of a human thighbone, a so-lame-it's-funny fake bed of hot coals you can "firewalk" across, a goofy fake cemetery with a well-done disappearing-man illusion, and the world's biggest boot. The Spacewalk maze near the exit is actually the scariest and most disorienting part of the whole place. Many people have to be dragged into it. There's chintzy stuff here, too, but that's what gives museums like this their charm.

The Sylvia Beach Hotel: 267 Northwest Cliff Street, overlooking the beach. Room rates: $40–$90. Many rooms are open to view, free, in the early afternoon. Phone: (503) 265-5428.

We'll be the first to admit that this is a darned clever idea (though a tad pretentious): Renovate a rundown beach hotel, name it after someone with "beach" in her name, and then take the literary theme and run with it. Each of the 20 guest rooms is named for a famous person and decorated accordingly. To wit: The Robert Louis Stevenson room sports a steamer trunk; the Tennessee Williams room has a mosquito-netting-draped bed and a glass menagerie; the Poe room has red-flowered black wallpaper, a stuffed raven, and even a scary pendulum; the Dr. Seuss room has funny hats. Other rooms are dedicated to Gertrude Stein, Colette, Oscar Wilde, and

Emily Dickinson. Allusions and adulation are as thick and relentless here as *The Tempest* itself, and we found ourselves at last giggling uncontrollably, calling the place the Saliva Bleach Motel, and acting as defiantly illiterate as possible.

The Waxworks: Mariner Square, 250 Southwest Bay Boulevard. Open in summer, daily, 9 A.M.–8 P.M.; other times, daily, 10 A.M.–5 P.M. Admission: $4; students 12–17, $3; children 5–11, $2; children under 5, free. Phone: (503) 265-2206.

Newport has three tacky tourist attractions clustered at the end of Bay Boulevard. The two listed here are worth a look, if only to marvel at the depths to which American taste can plunge. The third, Undersea Gardens, should be avoided at all costs, as it consists of one murky, lamely stocked aquarium attached to an overpriced gift shop. At the waxworks you at least get your money's worth. Gawk at the naked breasts of a lady Bigfoot; stagger across a shaky wooden bridge; let Medusa turn *you* to wax. A dimly lit "cabaret" has wax parodies of celebrities in every seat. *Star Wars, M.A.S.H.,* and *Raiders of the Lost Ark* go into the cultural jumble for good measure. The figures move and make sounds, too.

Zig Zag Zoo: 2640 Southwest Abalone Street in the town of South Beach, which is just south of Newport Bridge. If you're coming from the north, look for a crazily decorated mobile home on the west side and take the first exit after the bridge; from the south, exit left just before the bridge. Always visible. Admission: free.

Loran Finch used to wander the Oregon beaches, picking up a piece of driftwood here, another piece there. Bit by bit, he transformed the yard of his mobile home into Zig Zag Zoo, a hallucinatory flotsam and jetsam extravaganza. Painted driftwood faces leer from every angle. A fence made of nets, floats, and oars lines one side of the property. A plaster Snow White huddles conspiratorially with four of her dwarves; a fifth sits on a toilet nearby. Pieces of driftwood sport names, such as Fresno, Bob Hope, and Holy Cow—Moo! An antler lies entombed in a crab trap. A cement frog squats in a frisbee. A wishing-well milk can has a sign reading "Pennies for paint." It's a plea so sincere that you can't help but toss a few coins in the can.

PORTLAND

The American Advertising Museum: 9 NW 2nd Avenue, between Burnside and Couch. Museum is on second floor. Open Wednesday–Friday, 11 A.M.–5 P.M.; Saturday and Sunday, noon–5 P.M. Closed Monday–Tuesday. Admission: $1.50; children under 12, free. Phone: (503) 226-0000.

We bet you've eaten a lot of Froot Loops in your life. And why have you eaten them? Because you liked the toucan. Admit it. The world's most effective ad campaigns are examined at this slick, all-moving-all-talking museum. You'll see antique sandwich boards; videos; props used in TV commercials; fountain pens imprinted with catchy slogans; and memorabilia advertising Coca-Cola, Morton Salt, and other venerable American money-makers. A pictorial timeline traces the evolution of advertising gimmicks, and Burma Shave placards shout, "Statistics prove/near and far/that folks/who drive like crazy/...are!" You'll come out of here programmed to buy everything in the world.

Bizarre Storefront: 219 SW Ankeny, near 2nd Avenue, two blocks south of Burnside Street near downtown. Always visible.

"World's Cheapest Psychic 24 Hour 25¢ Cheap Where's the Art!!" announces the sign in front of this storefront-without-a-store. A homemade vending machine is installed in the window. Deposit your quarter; press your "favorite" button (many colors to choose from). Watch as a women's bowling trophy selects a prize for you, which then drops through a hole cut into the door. We can't tell you what kind of prizes pop out since we never got one. The machine was out of order when we visited. Multicolored American cultural detritus surrounds the dysfunctional vending device. What's it all mean? It means "Look at me—I'm an artist!" That's what it means.

Carousel Museum: 830 NE Holiday, at 8th Avenue NE. Open daily, 11 A.M.–5 P.M. Phone: (503) 235-2252.

A Victorian absinthe tippler's reverie comes to life as carved carousel lions, tigers, elephants, dogs, bulls, and even a mighty elk stand poised, waiting to run madly away. Also here, for the purist, are carousel horses of every color, as well as old carousel organs. Right next door is the museum's prized possession, a glorious carousel, which you can ride for 75¢.

Elephant Museum: in the extreme rear of Washington Park Zoo, west of downtown in Washington Park. Take Tri-Met bus 63 from downtown. Open daily, 9:30 A.M.–dusk. Admission: $2.50; children, $1.25. Phone: (503) 226-1561.

A huge mastodon overlooks elephant artworks (including Dalí originals and tribal masks), elephant trainers' spangly costumes, and elephant saddles. Every aspect of elephants shows up here—even elephant jokes and copies of *Babar the Elephant*. Exhibits explore Elephants at Work, Elephants in Literature, Elephants in Politics, and Elephants at War. Don't miss the elephanticycle or the elaborate miniature diorama showing elephants fighting alongside Hannibal in the Second Punic War. Most poignant of all is a discussion of the ivory trade.

Giant Heart: in the field to the right of the Oregon Museum of Science and Industry, at 4015 SW Canyon Road, in Washington Park next to the zoo. Take Tri-Met bus 63 from downtown. Always open. Admission: free. Phone: (503) 222-2828.

"Don't look now, Martha, but we're being attacked by a giant heart!" B-boom, b-boom, B-BOOM, B-BOOM... The Heart That Ate Portland! This 12-foot-tall, anatomically perfect, fiberglass human heart served its time as a museum demonstration exhibit and has now

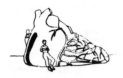

been put out to pasture in the field next to the museum. Blue and red veins, arteries, and mystery tubes go all over. A passageway leads into the right atrium.

Pretend you're a little blood cell and walk over to the left atrium. Now you're circulating!

Humane Society Tours: 1067 NE Columbia Boulevard, one mile east of Highway 5 at the Columbia Boulevard exit. Open Monday–Saturday, 9 A.M.–noon and 1–5 P.M.; Sunday, 10:30 A.M.–noon and 1–5 P.M. Ask for a free, self-guided tour map. Admission: free. Phone: (503) 285-0641.

The nation's second-oldest pet cemetery awaits you, brimming with over 2,000 graves. Most famous of these belongs to Bobby, the Oregon dog who walked thousands of miles in search of his owners. (Rin Tin Tin attended Bobby's funeral. Bobby's own doghouse marks his grave.) Also on the tour you'll see kennels, deluxe catteries, and a barnyard whose residents—a pig, lamb, cow, horse, burro, and others—were rejected by their former owners. Don't miss the marble drinking fountain for horses (once these were a common sight in downtown Portland) and the flagpole dedicated to K-9 Corps war casualties.

Mill Ends Park: in the center of the intersection of SW Front and Taylor, next to the waterfront park. Always visible.

Thick with foliage and protected by a fearsome fence, this majestic park covers a vast 452.16 square inches. Grandly it dominates the two-foot-square cement divider at Front and Taylor. Mill Ends Park, universally recognized as the world's smallest park, was dreamed up by a newspaper columnist on a slow news day. The park's single red geranium has played host to both weddings and car accidents—so don't get the idea that the Mill Ends Park ranger has a cushy job.

Portland Police Museum: 1111 SW 2nd Avenue, in the Justice Center Building, on the 16th floor, room 1682. Open Tuesday–Friday, 10 A.M.–3 P.M. Admission: free. Phone: (503) 796-3019.

You've probably never heard of Portland's most gruesome mass murderer, Earle Nelson, "The Gorilla Man." Neither did we, until we saw a graphic exhibit about him at the Portland Police Museum. Just as scary, but in a different way, is the bizarre Will West Case, in which a convicted murderer and an innocent man had the same name, height, arm span, head size, ear size, foot size, cheek width, home state, level of education, and life story, not to mention looking like clones of one another. A less-than-infallible police identification system justified the arrest of the wrong one. Also fascinating here is the homemade weapons exhibit, including guns made from scratch in prison. Keep an eye peeled for the hilariously outdated display on narcotics and their slang names.

The Sanctuary of Our Sorrowful Mother: 8840 NE Skidmore (corner of Sandy Boulevard and NE 85th). From downtown, take Tri-Met bus 12. Grounds are open Monday–Friday, 9 A.M.–5:30 P.M.; Saturday and Sunday, 9 A.M.–6:30 P.M. Gift shop and elevator open 10 A.M.–4

P.M. Admission: lower level is free, but donations are welcomed. Elevator to upper level: $2; seniors and children 6–18, $1; children under 6, free. Phone: (503) 254-7371.

You'd expect to find this kind of thing in Europe, where the devout have more space, more time, and more company. These 64 acres of landscaped woodland are dedicated to peace, quiet, meditation, and the Virgin Mary, whom the sourpuss Servite Order, who runs the place, calls "Our Sorrowful Mother." The focal point is The Grotto, a 30-by-50-foot cavern hewn out of a solid stone cliff. It is peopled with a marble Pietà and two sympathetic bronze angels bearing torches. Ivy and ferns tumble about the grotto. And don't miss the shrine of St. Peregrine, "the Cancer Saint" (the disease—not the zodiac sign).

PORT ORFORD
(28 miles north of Gold Beach)

Oregon Coast Llamas: 46968 Highway 101, 11 miles north of town in an unincorporated area called Denmark. Open daylight hours. Admission: free. Phone: (503) 348-2267.

Okay, you're striding along a golden southern Oregon beach, and suddenly you need an instant llama fix. What to do? The 11 critters on this ranch are more than willing to oblige, with quivering noses and unruffled stares.

Prehistoric Gardens: 12 miles south of town on Highway 101, west side of the road. Official address is 36848 Highway 101 South. Open daily, 8 A.M.–dusk. Admission: $3.50; students 12–18, $3; children 5–11, $2; children under 5, free. Phone: (503) 332-4463.

Though a few of these multicolored monsters wear a proper saurian scowl, most seem to be slyly grinning or letting out hearty guffaws. From the looks of this place, dinosaurs must have laughed themselves into extinction. T. rex, with a gleaming yellow tummy, greets you in the parking lot; a curious allosaurus peeks over the trees to see who's coming to visit. Paths through an Oregon-style rain forest lead to the other dinosaurs. Each has an explanatory sign. The bug-eyed, cackling triceratops is our personal favorite.

Sand Castle Contest: July 4. Starts at 9 A.M.; judging around noon. Port Beach, Port Orford Dock Road. For more information, call (503) 332-8055.

Build, sculpt, pile, scrape, dig, and mold your way to fame on the sands of Port Orford. The contest is part of a multifaceted July 4 Jubilee, and it has various age categories so that the little 'uns can have a fighting chance.

REDMOND

Llamas and More: 6615 Southwest McVey, five miles south of town. Visits by appointment only. Admission: free. Phone: (503) 548-5821.

"Llamas are here to stay!" proclaim the owners of this farm, who encourage visitors to meet and pet their 18 sloe-eyed specimens. Also raised here are pheasants, swans, and long-haired rabbits. Each visitor receives a free llama booklet and, if so moved, may purchase llama stationery, llama refrigerator magnets, and suchlike.

Operation Santa Claus: 4355 West Highway 126, two miles west of town. Open daily, dawn–dusk. Admission: free, but donations are accepted. Phone: (503) 548-8910.

Here at the world's largest commercial reindeer ranch, you'll learn the crucial reindeer facts that Santa himself memorized long ago: what they eat, what they do, how their antlers grow, and more. The best time to visit is in the early morning or early evening, when the 99 reindeer are fed and the babies are mostly out in the open. But never, no matter when you visit, will you see them fly. They just don't do that for strangers.

Petersen Rock Gardens: 7930 Southwest 77th Street, off Highway 97, 7½ miles south of Redmond and ten miles north of Bend. (Follow the signs.) Open in summer, daily, 7 A.M.–9 P.M.; in winter, daily, 7 A.M.–dusk. Admission to Rock Gardens: $1.50; children, 6–16, 50¢; children under 6, free. Admission to Fluorescent Room: 25¢; children, 10¢. Phone: (503) 382-5574.

In 1935, Danish immigrant Rasmus Petersen decided to wage war on the piles of rock that lay all over his farm and rendered much of his land unhoeable. Petersen collected the offending members, and slowly and patiently built them into scale-model castles, U.S. government buildings, churches, ponds, and bridges. Today you can see four acres' worth of Petersen's neat, symmetrical renderings: The Statue of Liberty, Independence Hall, and all your other old favorites are here. A rock and mineral museum on the property features the Fluorescent Room, in which little bridges and castles made of zinc, tungsten, uranium, and manganese glow in the dark.

ROCKAWAY
(14 miles north of Tillamook)

Sand Sculpture Contest: a low-tide Saturday in late June (varies). On the beach opposite the State Wayside, off Highway 101. For current date and other information, call (503) 355-8282 or (503) 355-8170.

Each contestant gets a generous 20-by-20-foot plot of sand to work with. Past winners have created a life-size (?) unicorn and an equally life-size (?) sea serpent. No sand castles are allowed—absolutely none.

ROGUE RIVER
(Eight miles east of Grants Pass)

National Rooster Crowing Contest: the last Saturday in June, 2:30 P.M.; at the Elementary School playground, on Pine Street. For more information, call (503) 582-0242.

How many times can your rooster crow in half an hour? Redland Red managed 48 crows in 1987, enough to win his owner a hefty sum. White Lightning, the all-time champion, pierced the air 112 times in 1978. Proud rooster owners descend on Rogue River every summer, birds in hand, eager to prove their superiority. The funniest part is not the birds but the owners, who resort to desperate tactics to get their cocks in the mood.

SALEM

Antique Valentine Display: the Sunday closest to Valentine's Day, noon–4:30 P.M. Deepwood Mansion, 1116 Mission Street Southeast (at 12th Street). Take Cherriots bus 15 from downtown. Admission: $2; seniors and students, $1.50; children, 75¢. Phone: (503) 363-1825.

This stately Queen Anne house, with its famous stained-glass windows, is a perfect setting for the frilly flock of Victorian valentine cards that are exhibited here once a year. The valentines, which once belonged to an old Salem family, include many that are well over 100 years old. Hearts, flowers, cupids, and lace—after this you'll say phooey to modern love.

Enchanted Forest: 8462 Enchanted Way SE, seven miles south of Salem in Turner; take exit 248 off Highway 5 and go south on Enchanted Way. Open March 15– September, daily, 9:30 A.M.–6 P.M. Admission: $3.50; children 3–12, $3; children under 3, free. Haunted house: 50¢; bobsled, 75¢. Phone: (503) 363-3060 or (503) 371-4242.

Walt Disney was a wimp. Did he build Disneyland all by himself, brick by brick, nail by nail? Of course not, you say. He'd have to be nuts to do that. Ah, but up here in Oregon a man did what Disney dared not do: He designed and built his own amusement park all alone, with no outside help. For seven years, Roger Tofte worked like a man possessed and opened Enchanted Forest to the public in 1971. It's still growing. Today, you can walk into the witch's head, two stories of pure ugliness. Have a reunion with the denizens of fairy tales: the Old Lady's Shoe, the crooked man and his crooked house, the seven dwarves' cottage, and others. There's also a false-front Western town (Tofteville, of course), an English Village, Alice-in-Wonderland vignettes, and much more.

SAND LAKE
(14 miles southwest of Tillamook)

William Ward's Carved Bears: 7575 Galloway Road. When you arrive in Sand Lake, turn west at Sand Lake Grocery. After 1½ miles, go slow and look for a mailbox on the left (south) side of the road, at the two-mile point. There's no name or number on the box, but go up the driveway and look for bears in the yard. Don't disturb the occupants of the house; just stroll around. If you get lost, ask for directions at Sand Lake Grocery; the owner is Ward's daughter. Visible anytime. Admission: free. Phone (Sand Lake Grocery, open 8 A.M.–8 P.M.): (503) 965-6152.

William Ward used to be a hunter, but after a bear almost killed his dog, he had a change of heart about bears. He stopped shooting them and started sculpting them. Ward is now in that great Chain-Saw Carving Hall of Fame in the sky, yet his wooden bears remain. Did you know Smokey the Bear has a wife? Well, he does, and she's captured here forever in wood. A minister bear preaches to his ursine flock: "Don't eat innocent humans, my children." Bears aren't the whole story here; you'll also see big owls, eagles, Abe Lincoln, a totem pole, and the ubiquitous Bigfoot.

SEAL ROCK
(Five miles north of Waldport, on the coast)

Sea Gulch: on Highway 101 at the north end of the tiny town of Seal Rock on the east side of the road. You can't miss it. Open in summer, daily, 8 A.M.–7 P.M.; in winter, daily, 8 A.M.–dusk. Admission: $3.50; seniors, $2.50; children, $2; children under 5, free. Phone: (503) 563-2520 or (503) 563-2727.

Chain-saw carving is to sculpture what industrial music is to the concerto. And there's no better introduction to the world of chain-saw art than Sea Gulch, a wild-west beach town in redwood. Owner Ray Kowalski hacks out comical carvings at a furious pace, and most of them end up on the Sea Gulch trail, a quarter-mile whirlwind of cowboys, Bigfeet, gnomes, humanoid bears, and visual puns. The theme is podunk western sarcasm, with a gaggle of storybook characters filling out the collection. Don't miss the towering Horizontal Tree Farm.

SHERWOOD
(16 miles southwest of Portland)

Robin Hood Festival: third weekend in July. Events take place all over town. Saturday-morning costume parade travels down North Sherwood Boulevard, starting at 10 A.M. For more information, call (503) 625-6751.

A shameless example of the old capitalize-on-your-own-name trick, but the medieval costumes are fun. Craft and food booths spring up all over town for the occasion, and the high point is an archery competition—the results of which are annually pitted against those of a simultaneous shoot-off in Nottingham, England.

SILVERTON
(12 miles northeast of Salem)

Davenport Races: first Saturday in August, 1 P.M., on Main Street. Admission: free. For more information, call (503) 873-5615.

You mean—couches? That's right. No beer-bellies slouched in front of the TV in this town. Becostumed local folk equip their sofas with racing wheels and wild decorations and ride them crazily down the street in a series of competitions leading to the Davenport championships. It's all a pun based on the name of Homer Davenport, a favorite native-son political cartoonist.

SWEET HOME
(27 miles southeast of Albany)

White's Electronics Museum: 1011 Pleasant Valley Road, next to the front office of White's Electronics Company. Open Monday–Friday, 7:30 A.M.–4:30 P.M. Admission: free. Phone: (503) 367-2138.

White's manufactures metal detectors: the treasure hunter's beeping, buzzing, flat-faced answer to bloodhounds. On display at the museum is bounty actually found with the help of metal detectors: coins, bullets, bottles, even Civil War relics. Especially mouth-watering is the collection of valuable objects that the company's founders discovered in a sunken Spanish ship off the Atlantic coast. Also note the vintage 1940s geiger counters and early metal detectors.

TILLAMOOK

The Octopus Tree: in Cape Meares State Park, ten miles west of Tillamook on the Three Capes Scenic Drive. Tree is just south of the parking lot, on the hiking trail. Visible anytime. Admission: free. Phone: (503) 842-7525.

Although this big Sitka spruce won't actually thrust out tentacled limbs and wrestle you to the ground, it *is* strange looking. Even Robert Ripley thought so. Instead of a thick, vertical main trunk, the Octopus Tree has several five-foot-thick branches emerging from the ground, arching out horizontally, and then reaching straight for the sky. These limbs resemble canoes; hence the local legend that ancient natives buried their chiefs beside the tree and stuck the dead men's boats on the branches.

Pig 'n' Ford Races: second weekend in August. Two races each on Thursday, Friday, and Saturday, starting at 4:30 P.M. Part of the Tillamook County Fair at the Tillamook Fairgrounds, east side of town. Admission to fair: $4; children, $1. Phone: (503) 842-7525.

Let's get this straight: Five men each dash to grab a wriggling, squealing pig from a pen. Clutching their prey, they jump into roofless Model T Fords (which the men must crank-start by hand), drive around a muddy track, stop, exchange their pigs for new ones, hand-crank their Model Ts again, and so on. This has some historical significance, but do you really want to know what it is? And the race is funny. Funny as heck. Especially when the pigs break free and run oinking to freedom. The climactic championship race is on Saturday evening.

VIDA

(27 miles east of Eugene)

House of Horses: 45834 McKenzie Highway, at the 27.5 milepost, one-half mile east of Vida. Open Monday–Thursday, 10 A.M.–4 P.M.; Friday, 10 A.M.–noon. Closed Saturday–Sunday. Admission: $1; children, 50¢. Babies and toddlers not admitted. Phone: (503) 896-3105.

Martha Shelley, well past 90 but still a whittler supreme, created rows of elaborate dioramas depicting her own family riding, raising, training, and otherwise interacting with horses. Since 1957, she has filled the museum with her own carvings, as well as paintings, silhouettes, and sketches of horses in every posture and mood.

WALDPORT

Beachcomber Days: third weekend in June. Slug races: Saturday in the parking lot of Alsea River Cable Company. Crab races: Saturday in front of Crab Manufacturing Company, on the bay front. Keg toss: Saturday, parking lot of Old Town Tavern. Sand castle contest: Sunday, on the waterfront at Old Town. Slug and crab rental: 50¢. For more information, call (503) 563-4859.

Surely this is what Robinson Crusoe, world's greatest beachcomber, would have wanted to see: little beachcomber children tormenting slugs and crabs in the name of competition, their big strong beachcomber daddies hurling beer kegs around in a parking lot.... Well, he would have liked the sand castle contest. Maybe.

WILSONVILLE
(18 miles south of Portland)

Grove of the States: at the Baldock Safety Rest Area, south of Wilsonville off exit 282 of Highway 5, on the west side of the highway. Visible anytime. Admission: free.

Every state has its own official bird, flower, song, and tree. But you can never see them all in one place. Except here. The trees, at least. A map at the entrance to the trail shows where each tree is, and a plaque at each tree gives the state-by-state lowdown. Gee, we'd never even heard of the eastern redbud, and it's the Oklahoma state tree. You learn something new every day.

WASHINGTON

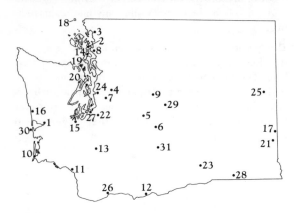

Legend:
1. Aberdeen
2. Anacortes
3. Bellingham
4. Carnation
5. Cle Elum
6. Ellensburg
7. Issaquah
8. La Conner
9. Leavenworth
10. Long Beach
11. Longview
12. Maryhill
13. Morton
14. Oak Harbor
15. Olympia
16. Pacific Beach
17. Palouse
18. Point Roberts
19. Port Townsend
20. Poulsbo
21. Pullman
22. Puyallup
23. Richland
24. Seattle
25. Spokane
26. Stevenson
27. Tacoma
28. Walla Walla
29. Wenatchee
30. Westport
31. Yakima

Washingtonians like to say they live in "Washington, *the state.*" It's a gently sarcastic prod, a wisecracking way of tapping the world on the shoulder and murmuring, "Hey. Turn around."

It *is* unsettling to live in a country that has two Washingtons. The eastern one, small as it is, gets all the headlines. And yet the western one has the world's largest rosary collection. The world's smallest shrunken head. The world's first Skid Row, even.

You've heard of Washington's prized apples. But what of Washington's prized onions, the big 20-inchers that locals lob in Walla Walla's annual onion shot-put championship?

You're looking for filibusters? The Malaysian Embassy? John Wilkes Booth? Go east, young man.

ANACORTES

Causland Park Rockery: on 8th Street between M and N Avenues, north end of town. Open daily, 10 A.M.–6 P.M. Admission: free. Phone: (206) 293-4541.

Harry Causland was an Anacortes man killed while helping his comrades on a French battlefield during WWI. In honor of him and other local war dead, the city commissioned this whimsical yet serene mosaic park. French artist Jean Lepage (inspired by Spanish whimsy-master Antonio Gaudí) collected thousands of stones on beaches in the San Juan Islands area: red, brown, gray, yellow, black, white. He fashioned them into free-form walls, mounds, and archways, mosaicked with stars, pinwheels, and other shapes. It's a relief to see a war memorial that is, in effect, so peaceful.

BIRCH BAY
(20 miles northwest of Bellingham)

Sand Castle Contest: third Saturday in July, at the Birch Bay Beach in front of the Sea Links Restaurant. Construction begins at noon; judging is at 4 P.M. Phone: (206) 371-2070.

Part of Birch Bay's mid-July Discovery Days festival, this contest has categories for both sand castles and sand sculptures, adults' and children's divisions, and even cash prizes.

BONNEY LAKE
(16 miles southeast of Tacoma)

Mudflat Golf Tournament: a Saturday, usually in March, 9 A.M. South end of Lake Tapps, at Allen York Park, West Tapps Highway and Bonney Lake Boulevard. From Highway 410E, take the Tapps Lake Recreation Area turnoff. For current date and other information, call (206) 862-7051.

Every spring, the local utility company plays God and lowers the level of Lake Tapps, which is more a reservoir than a lake. Like opportunistic children around a broken fire hydrant, the locals gleefully turn the resultant knee-deep mudflat into an 18-hole golf course. Golfers arrive dressed as executives, cartoon characters, babies—anything. Prizes go to the golfer with the lowest score, the one with the highest score, the one with the muddiest costume, and the one with the cleanest costume.

CARNATION
(26 miles east of Seattle)

Camlann Medieval Faire: From Carnation, go two miles north on Highway 203 to the Stillwater Store. Turn right at the store and go one mile to the faire entrance. Open mid-July to late August, Saturday–Sunday, 11 A.M. –6 P.M. Admission: $7; seniors and children 7–12, $3; children under 7, free. Phone: (206) 788-1945.

What's the difference between a Renaissance faire and a medieval faire? About 200 years, forsooth, and don't you forget it. At Camlann (named after the site of King Arthur's last battle), the year is 1376—a moment in the last flowering of feudalism. In a tranquil wood, visitors mingle with fustian-clad craftspeople, knights in armor, ladies in finery, fire-swallowing jugglers, bawdy lute players, wisecracking tightrope walkers, and moralistic puppeteers. It's a careful and unaggressive kind of time tunnel. Visitors are encouraged to arrive in costume. You can also rent medieval garb at the faire.

Camlann Medieval Feasts: last two Saturdays of the Camlann Medieval Faire. Dinner is served around 6:30 P.M. For directions, see previous entry. Admission: $30 (includes admission to faire). Phone: (206) 788-1945.

Roste Fyssh is one of the dozen 14th-century delicacies that costumed servers place before you with great fanfare. Prepare your 20th-century stomach for *farced byrdes* (stuffed fowl), *farced funges* (stuffed mushrooms), *ypocras* (hot spiced wine), meat-and-berry pie, roast pork in boar's-tail sauce, and more. Minstrels accompany the meal, but for authenticity's sake, plates and utensils do not.

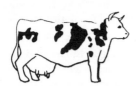

Carnation Research Farm: 28901 NE Carnation Farm Road. From the town of Carnation, go one mile north to the Carnation Farm turnoff; then go 2½ miles west to the farm. Open Monday–Saturday, 10 A.M.–3 P.M. Admission: free. Phone: (206) 788-1511. Pick up a free, self-guiding tour map at the front office.

At the entrance, pay your respects to the late Segis Pietertje Prospect, queen of cows, who yielded virtual oceans of milk in her lifetime. This statue is allegedly the first one ever erected in honor of a moo-cow. A tour of the farm includes visits to the milking carousel, the calf nursery, and the formal gardens.

CASHMERE
(12 miles northwest of Wenatchee)

Liberty Orchards Company, Inc.: 117 Mission Street (at Woodring), just off Highway 2. Tours given daily in summer, 8 A.M.–5 P.M.; in winter, Monday–Friday, 8 A.M.–4 P.M. Admission: free. Phone: (509) 782-2191.

Whether or not you actually like pectin and powdered sugar, you have to admit that Aplets and Cotlets are the cutest names in the whole candy kingdom. A knowledgeable guide leads you through the kitchens where these cubist treats are manufactured and then tempts you with free samples.

CLE ELUM

Telephone Museum: 221 East 1st Street. Open Tuesday–Friday, 10 A.M.–4 P.M.; Saturday–Sunday, noon–4 P.M. Admission: voluntary donation. Phone: (509) 674-5958.

The big switchboards have stood here, lonely and silent, ever since the town's three full-time human operators were traded for a direct-dial phone system in 1966. Also here are dozens of vintage phones.

COPALIS BEACH
(25 miles northwest of Aberdeen, on the coast)

Sand Sculpture Contest: usually the Saturday of July 4 weekend. Building starts at 11 A.M., judging at 2 P.M. On the Benner Gap Road section of Copalis Beach, in front of the town. For more information, call (206) 289-4552.

Five hundred people show up to watch as oceanic shoreline environmental sculptors impose their wills on helpless but free-spirited grains of sand.

DUPONT
(15 miles south of Tacoma)

Dupont Historical Museum: 207 Barksdale Avenue in Dupont, which is next to Fort Lewis; take exit 119 to the north side of Highway 5. Open May–August, Wednesday, 7–9 P.M., and Sunday, 1–4 P.M.; September–April, Sunday, 1–4 P.M. only. Admission: free. Phone: (206) 964-8895 or (206) 964-2399.

Formerly called Dupont Powderworks, this was a company town for a dynamite factory owned by the giant chemical corporation Dupont. Residents had only one occupation: making dynamite. The museum, housed in the old butcher shop (is there a hint of symbolism here?), has dynamite casings, machines for packing gunpowder, special non-spark-causing shovels, an exhibit on the dynamite assembly line, and plenty of photos, as well as clothing worn by the workers. Hey—DON'T LIGHT THAT MATCH! Just kidding. There's no gunpowder left in this town. Or so they say.

EATONVILLE
(30 miles south of Tacoma)

Slug Festival: usually the second weekend in July, with races at 12:30 and 3 P.M. on Saturday and Sunday. Northwest Trek Wildlife Park, six miles north of Eatonville on Highway 161 (look for the signs). Admission: $5.50; children 5–17, $3; seniors, $4; children 3–4, $1. Phone: (206) 847-1901 or (206) 847-1903.

Yet another example of the mollusk mania that's sweeping the Northwest: This one is a high-class affair, with sophisticated timing devices for the speeding slugs and special stables from which you rent them. Knowledgeable wildlife experts conduct a brutal slug trivia contest. The emphasis here is on animal education, not animal exploitation.

EDMONDS
(Ten miles north of Seattle)

Cannonball and Bellyflop Contest: second Thursday in July, 7 P.M. Yost Park Pool, 96th and Bowdoin. For more information, call (206) 775-2645 or (206) 775-2525.

Cannonballs and bellyflops are to diving what cotton candy and Ripple are to eating. Various age groups compete throughout the evening. Whereas cannonballers are judged on the size of their splashes, the intrepid, insane bellyfloppers deserve a medal for bravery: They *must* land belly first, and they are judged on the sharpness of their slap. Esther Williams, run and hide.

ELLENSBURG

Dick and Jane's Spot: 101 North Pearl Street (at 1st Avenue), across the street from the police station. Always visible from the sidewalk; do not enter the yard, as it is private property. For more information, call the Chamber of Commerce at (509) 925-3137.

Such a restrained, tactful name for such a manic place. Dick Elliot and Jane Orleman, once mild-mannered artists, went off the deep end around 1980 and unleashed their new-found creative energy on their house and yard. The primary units of expression here are traffic reflectors and bottle caps. These are nailed and stuck in great shiny profusion to every available surface. Bold colors confront you on all sides, and glittering homemade windmills spin madly. A gigantic hand emerges from the front of the house, as humanoid figures made of poles and car parts accost the visitor. Thirty artists have contributed to the yard, which is still constantly evolving.

ELMA
(27 miles west of Olympia)

The Elma Slug Festival: usually the last weekend in July. Slug races: Friday afternoon and Saturday late morning and afternoon; championship, Saturday afternoon. Slug parade: Saturday at noon. All races are on the stage set up in the center of town. Phone: (206) 482-2212.

This is Washington's undisputed original slug festival. The town's mascot, Thelma the Elma Slug, rides through the streets on a huge float during the slug parade. Highlights are the blindingly slow slug races, with a series of adults' and children's preliminaries leading up to the slug championships Saturday around 4 P.M.

FAIRHAVEN
(A suburb of Bellingham)

Slug Race: the first Sunday after Labor Day, 3 P.M., at the gazebo at 12th Street and Harris Avenue. Take exit 250 from Highway 5. For more information, call (206) 671-7573.

Iridescent slime trails glint seductively in the sun as dozens of children race their favorite slugs. They urge the unwitting animals along with fragrant marigolds and bad puns ("Slug it out!"). The slugs measure about four inches; the racetrack measures 18 inches. The slug that "runs" the farthest in three minutes is the winnah.

FALL CITY
(20 miles east of Seattle)

Llama Fest: the weekend nearest July 4. The Herbfarm: From Seattle, take Highway 90 east and get off at exit 22. Go north three miles; where the road forks, go left over a green bridge. Keep going until you reach a stop sign. The Herbfarm is across the street. For more information, call (206) 784-2222.

Kids (60 pounds and under) get to ride a saddled llama. Performers sing and tell stories about llamas. Craftspeople show how to spin llama wool into useful items. Experts reveal llama-packing tips. The llamas themselves dash around an obstacle course to demonstrate their agility. Okay, okay. Now, when are they gonna have one of these shindigs for dugongs?

GRAYLAND
(Seven miles south of Westport)

Twin Harbors Driftwood Show: third weekend in March. For more information, call (206) 267-7671.

This here is prime beachcombing territory. All sorts of curious objects have been known to turn up on Washington beaches after traveling halfway around the world on strong ocean currents. At this beachcombers' art show and contest, you'll see carved driftwood, cleverly painted kelp, and much surprising flotsam.

ISSAQUAH

Boehm's Candy Tours and Edelweiss Chalet: 255 Northeast Gilman Boulevard, off Front Street. Take exit 17 off Highway 90. Tours by appointment only. Admission: free. Phone: (206) 392-6652.

This is no ersatz Swiss chalet. It was built by a real Swiss person. The late Herr Boehm escaped Nazi-riddled Europe in 1940 and built himself the kind of house he had known and loved all his life. On the 40-minute tour, you'll see lots of Alpine artifacts, both folk art and fine art: beer steins, stained-glass windows, elk antlers, coats-of-arms. Downstairs, you can watch workers hand-dipping chocolates. Also on the property is Boehm's *kirch'l*, a replica of a 12th-century Swiss chapel.

KINGSTON
(Ten miles northeast of Poulsbo, on the Kitsap Peninsula)

Slug Race: July 4, usually in Kola Kole Park, but the location is subject to change. For more information, call (206) 297-3633.

This is a BYOS affair (Bring Your Own Slugs). The racetrack is a three-foot circle; the slugs are placed in the center, and the first one to make it to the edge is the winner. (In human society, the first one to make it to the edge is put in the asylum.) Slug experts offer this advice: Slugs love geraniums, so if you're playing to win, have a few of these on hand. Dangle them in front of your slug's—um—nose(?) and he'll be off and running like a greyhound after a mechanical rabbit.

LA CONNER

Tillinghast Seed Company Museum: corner of Morris and Maple, at the entrance to town. Open Monday–Saturday, 10 A.M.–5 P.M.; Sunday, noon–6 P.M. Admission: free. Phone: (206) 466-3329.

The artifacts here, culled from the attics of historic Tillinghast Seed Company, reveal the ins and outs of a century in the mail-order seed business—from its first sprouting all the way to its greatest flowering. On display are brilliant antique catalog covers and seed packets, seed bins, garden tools, and other equipment.

LANGLEY
(On the southern end of Whidbey Island)

Langley Mystery Weekend: a weekend in mid-February (varies). Game hours: Saturday–Sunday, 10 A.M.–5 P.M.; clues are distributed throughout the city. Admission: free. For current dates and location of Mystery Headquarters, call (206) 321-6765.

Hordes of tiptoeing Miss Marples and Father Browns descend on Langley to act out their detective fantasies.

The mystery is different every year. Would-be detectives collect clues at the scene of the crime and from "participating merchants." (This last phrase should tip you off that the whole affair is a ploy to get tourists into Langley in the off-season.) A play, performed Sunday evening, reenacts the crime and unravels the mystery. The player with the correct answer is announced and prizes are awarded. If you plan to participate, reserve a room well in advance.

LEAVENWORTH

Bavarian Ice Fest: Martin Luther King, Jr. weekend (mid-January). Snow sculpture contest: Saturday afternoon, Front Street. For more information, call (509) 548-5807.

When the people of Leavenworth say "Bavarian," they mean it. Or they think they do. Or they want you to think they do. Leavenworth has enough Teutonique-nouveau décor to send Hitler himself screaming down der street in agony. Still, snow sculpturing exhibitions are rare indeed, so try to grin und bear it. Last year's winning sculpture was a life-size snow-car.

LITTLEROCK
(12 miles south of Olympia)

Mima Mounds: Go south from Olympia on Highway 5, exit west at exit 95, go through Littlerock on Highway 121, and continue west on 128th Avenue SW; turn right on Waddell Creek Road until you come to the signposted entrance. Open daily, 9 A.M.–dusk; occasionally closed in bad weather. Admission: free. Phone: (206) 753-2449.

Rarely do you hear the words "Mima Mounds" without the word "mysterious" preceding them. Few geological oddities have undergone such intensive scientific scrutiny and yet remained unexplained. The Mima Mounds are just that—mounds. Bumps. Four hundred and forty-five acres of them, most around seven feet high and 30 feet across. The question is, where did they come from? Nobody knows, though the theories are as funny as they are numerous: giant gopher mounds, the results of postglacial freezing, an alien burial ground. We're currently leaning toward the "earth acne" theory. Don't forget your dowsing rod!

LONG BEACH

Marsh's Free Museum: 409 Pacific Highway 103, between 4th and 5th Streets. Open in summer, daily, 9 A.M.–10 P.M.; in winter, daily, 9 A.M.–6 P.M. Admission: free. Phone: (206) 642-2188.

Prime exotica, maritime gewgaws, arcade antiques, and choice beachcombing discoveries all await you here. A preserved two-headed pig has a tête-à-tête-à-tête-à-tête with a two-headed calf. Finds from West Coast shipwrecks include frying pans, life preservers, and hatch covers. Jake the Alligator Man, a retired sideshow curiosity, looks just as dubious now as he always did. Japanese fishing floats, old mechanical music devices, a shrunken head...you get the idea.

Sand-Sations Sand Castle Contest: on a Saturday in mid- to late July, depending on the tides. Construction runs 10 A.M.–noon; judging is at 2 P.M., on the portion of beach next to the town of Long Beach. Turn west at Bolstad Street, which has the only stoplight in town. For more information, call (206) 642-2400.

Though this annual contest started as recently as 1985, it's already one of the big events on the sand castle circuit. Why? Try $1,500 in cash prizes, at least 10,000 spectators, and the world's longest beach. What sand sculptor could resist? Some of the coast's finest creations turn up here, both in the sand castle and sand sculpture categories.

LONGVIEW

Suspension Bridge for Squirrels: on Olympia Way. Visible anytime. For more information, call (206) 423-8400.

Forty years ago, Amos Peters' sons were sad. Too many squirrels were getting their furry little selves flattened as they tried to cross the road. The boys convinced their dad, a construction contractor, to build the squirrels their very own bridge. It's fastened to tall trees on either side, so the squirrels can scurry high over the road, instead of on it.

MARYHILL
(On the Columbia River, ten miles south of Goldendale)

Stonehenge Replica: just southeast of the intersection of Highways 97 and 14, overlooking the Columbia River. Follow the sign from the Highway 14 exit. Always open. Admission: free. For more information, call the Maryhill Museum at (509) 773-3733.

In England, Stonehenge is a prehistoric astronomic observatory, made of monoliths that were dragged great distances. In America, Stonehenge is a monument to the soldiers of WWI (built, oddly, before the war was over). It's made of poured cement. Sam Hill, the entrepreneur who built this Stonehenge, didn't know the original Stonehenge had anything to do with telling the time of the solstices or measuring changes in the sky, so he built his Stonehenge with no regard to its angle and orientation. Even so, this one's in much better shape than the original. At least we've got them beat on that count.

McCLEARY
(20 miles west of Olympia)

Bear Festival: third Saturday in July; downtown at the corner of 3rd and Simpson. Parade begins at noon. For more information, call (206) 495-3863.

There used to be lots of bears around McCleary. Now there aren't so many. There used to be lots of folks wearing bear suits at the Bear Festival. Now there aren't so many. There used to be lots of real bear meat in the bear stew they serve at the festival. Now there isn't so much. But there *is* some.

MOCLIPS
(35 miles northwest of Aberdeen, on the coast)

Kelpers' Parade: Labor Day Sunday, 11 A.M.–2 P.M. Begins in Moclips' town center and continues down Highway 109 2½ miles to Pacific Beach. Anyone can join. For more information, call (206) 289-4552.

This frantic Northwest traveling shindig is the only procession to out-doo dah the Doo Dah Parade. Sure, this one is smaller, but do they wrap themselves in kelp in Pasadena? We think not. Remember, though, the kelp theme is only an excuse to stage the parade, and the one stricture on behavior and dress is "the crazier the better." That's in the *rules*. Prizes are doled out for best costumes.

MORTON
(55 miles south of Tacoma)

National Lawnmower Racing Championships: second Friday in August, 6 or 7 P.M. Part of the Morton Loggers' Jubilee, in the Jubilee Arena, east side of town. For more information, call (206) 498-5250.

"**B**rakes are legal, but not mandatory" states the official rule book for the lawnmower championships. And that about sums up the whole attitude of the contestants. We aren't talking about your standard hand-pushed lawnmowers, the kind used for cutting wimpy little blades of grass. No, these are sit-down, eight-horsepower, blades-removed, full-blown racing mowers. They're capable of speeds of up to a lawn-obliterating 35 mph. Tight turns, wrecks, and a screaming, frenzied crowd keep your heart pounding and your mind blank. "Mow, man, mow!"

OAK HARBOR
(On Whidbey Island)

Holland Happening: last weekend in April. Events are centered around Oak Harbor High School, corner of 700 Avenue and Heller Road, west of downtown. For more information, call (206) 675-3535.

Dutch immigrants came to Oak Harbor in the 1890s, and the town celebrates its heritage every year with wooden shoes, folk dancing, and demonstrations by the local keeshond club. (Keeshonds are the Dutch national dog. At the festival you can buy sweaters woven from their hair.) Even Burger King jumps into the act, printing a Dutch translation for "Whopper" on the menu (made from 100 percent *puur rundvlees*, ya know). Food booths dish up such Dutch favorites as tostadas, teriyaki, tacos, and buffalo burgers.

OCEAN SHORES
(19 miles west of Aberdeen)

Beachcombers' Fun Days: first weekend in March. Ocean Shores Convention Center, Chance-a-la-Mer Street, downtown. Admission: $1. For more information, call (206) 289-2451 or (206) 249-4628.

What can you do with driftwood? You'd be surprised. Beachcombers from all over Washington's coast show off their wave-tossed treasures. Guest speakers lecture on beachcombing topics—such as what to do when you find a shipwreck—and judges award prizes to the best driftwood art. Besides driftwood, you can also see collections of Japanese fishing floats, old shoes, and other gifts from Poseidon.

ORTING
(18 miles southeast of Tacoma)

Beard Contest, Bed Race, and Potty-Chair Race: usually the last Saturday in September or the first Saturday in October (varies). All events take place on Washington Street. For current date and more information, call (206) 893-6050.

These high-class events are part of the month-long Red Hat Days, named after a type of red felt hunting hat that the locals wear at this time of year. Women decorate the hats by gluing tiny plastic deer, trees, and infinitesimal gun-toting hunters around the brim. Thus the mood is set. Beds rocket down the street as beards are judged on softness, length, and grooming. "Potty chairs" are toilets on wheels. The race is limited to fire fighters, whose idea it was in the first place. One fire fighter in full uniform "rides" the toilet, while another (also in uniform) pushes it, and so on down the street.

PALOUSE
(14 miles northeast of Pullman)

Palouse Newspaper and Print Museum: 108 East Main Street. Open Memorial Day–September 15, Saturday and Sunday, 1–4 P.M., and by appointment. Admission: free. For more information, call (509) 878-1678.

In the last 15 years, the newspaper world has undergone a revolution. Gone are the old printing presses and metal type; gone are handwritten notes; gone are typewriters; gone are green visors. Computers do it all now, from getting the news, to writing the story, to typesetting the paper. This museum is dedicated to preserving a way of life that has all but disappeared. A replica of an old print shop shows what an inky, exacting profession this must have been. Another mock-up shows an old newsroom. Old machinery and newspapers round out the museum.

POINT ROBERTS
(20 miles south of Vancouver, B.C.)

Geopolitical Anomaly: Go north from Blaine into Canada on Highway 99; then turn south at Delta, B.C., to Point Roberts.

When, in 1846, the eastern politicians established the U.S.-Canadian border, the last thing on their minds was Point Roberts. It wasn't until some time later that the southern five miles of the Canadian peninsula below Vancouver were found to lie south of the 49th parallel. Oops. Point Roberts became part of the United States and remains so to this day. But Point Roberts isn't connected to the rest of the country. It's surrounded by water on three sides, and by Canada on the other side. Drivers from Point Roberts have to cross the international boundary twice just to get to the rest of Washington. Various international agreements make life there a little easier. The Canadians don't seem to mind. In fact, they love the place.

PORT TOWNSEND

Bed Race and Beard Contest: third weekend in May. Bed race: Friday, 6 P.M., down Lawrence and Monroe Streets. Beard contest: Saturday, noon, Memorial Stadium. For more information, call (206) 385-2722.

The thoroughbred beds are lavishly decorated according to a different theme every year. "Oh sheet!" cry the losers, and "Bedder luck next time!" jeer the winners. Judges award prizes to the proud owners of the longest beard, scruffiest beard, and prettiest beard.

Kinetic Sculpture Race: usually in early October (varies). Starts at noon. The course runs throughout the city; finish line is usually at Washington and Madison Streets. For more information, call (206) 385-5628.

Do you fight fair and play to win? Then stay away from Port Townsend's Kinetic Sculpture Race. Similar events are good-natured affairs, with smiles for the weirdest entry and polite laughs at breakdowns and wrecks. But in Port Townsend, the term "sense of humor" is an understatement. The human-powered, moving "sculptures" are expected to float on the bay, bump along railroad tracks, slog through a swamp, and climb an impossibly steep hill. The official rules insist, "No flatulating during radio or

TV interviews" and "In case of sun, the race will be held anyway."

POULSBO
(15 miles north of Bremerton)

Skandia Midsommarfest: a Sunday in late June (varies). Frank Raab Park, southern edge of town. Parade and pole raising: 2 P.M. Admission: $5; children under 12, free. For current date and more information call (206) 779-4848.

That great pagan tradition of raising the Maypole has not been forgotten here in Washington's "Little Norway." Pole raising is the centerpiece of a festival that features hundreds of folk dancers and craftspeople—some of whom come all the way from Scandinavia. Sorry, no midnight sun.

Viking Fest: the weekend closest to May 17. Events are centered on the waterfront. For more information, call (206) 779-4848.

Poulsbo is called "Little Norway" because of its fjordlike appearance and its many Norwegian-American residents. Viking Fest celebrates Norway's independence from Sweden. Events include street dancing, food booths, and husky fellers in Viking costumes. Best of all is a lutefisk-eating contest, during which participants gobble bowls of pallid, lye-soaked cod.

PULLMAN

Mycological Herbarium: third floor, Edward Johnson Hall, in the agricultural complex on the east side of the Washington State University campus. Open Monday–Friday, 8 A.M.–5 P.M. Admission: free. Phone: (509) 335-3732.

Sixty-eight thousand specimens from all over the world are stored in cabinets. If you're into fungus, a faculty member will take specimens out and show them to you. Please—don't eat the fungus.

Veterinary Anatomy Museum: second floor, Wegner Hall, Washington State University campus. Open Monday–Friday, 8 A.M.–5 P.M. Admission: free. Phone: (509) 335-8212.

Porpoise bones await you at this educational museum, where freeze-dried muscles and other animal parts float in gleaming jars and where skulls grin good-naturedly at all who pass by. Mammals are the focus here: cows, dogs, horses—you get the idea.

PUYALLUP

"Daffodil 200" Bed Race: usually the fourth Saturday in July. Bed parade begins at 10 A.M.; race begins 11 A.M. Meridian Street. For more information, call (206) 845-6755.

Prizes go to the best-decorated bed as well as the fastest one. Each bed has four muscular types pushing it and one white-knuckled rider (usually female, for some reason) who shrieks in terror as the beds careen down the street.

RICHLAND

Ye Merrie Greenwood Faire: a weekend in mid-June; Saturday and Sunday, noon–7 P.M., in Howard Amon Park. Admission: $1.50. For current dates and other information, call (509) 946-3131 or (509) 783-7727.

In this festival's version of Shakespeare's time, all the world really *is* a stage. Six stages feature continuous rollicking entertainment, 16th-century style: Shakespearean playlets, Renaissance dancers, even "japers"—rough-and-tumble Renaissance comedians. A noble queen in full regal regalia strolls through the faire, as do jousters, knights, cowled "monks," magicians, peasants, and washerwomen.

ROCHE HARBOR
(On San Juan Island)

Tomb of John McMillin: take ferry to Friday Harbor; from there drive to Roche Harbor. Once there at the Hotel de Haro, walk on the path northeast past the chapel, pool, and cottages back to Roche Harbor Road; turn left past the cemetery and turn right on the dirt road. Signs point the way to the mausoleum (about 200 yards). If you want to skip the hotel, simply turn right when entering Friday Harbor before reaching the gate to the hotel. Always open. Admission: free. Phone: (206) 378-2155.

Like the Pharaohs, John McMillin, founder of a successful cement and lime company, was not satisfied with being the king of his company town. He built himself an elaborate tomb, a memorial for the ages. The centerpiece is a circular colonnade surrounding a limestone table and chairs. The tomb brims with symbolism, especially Masonic symbolism. A deliberately broken column represents death; the ring on top of the columns represents immortality; seven stair steps represent the seven liberal arts; and so on. The ashes of the entire McMillin family are contained in the bases of the chairs. (For a full explanation of the symbolism, pick up the booklet at the hotel.) And to think Mozart lies in a pauper's grave.

SEATTLE

Archie McPhee and Company: 3510 Stone Way N, two blocks north of Lake Union. Open Monday–Thursday, 10 A.M.–5:30 P.M.; Friday, 10 A.M.–6 P.M.; Saturday, 10 A.M.–5 P.M. Admission: free. Phone: (206) 547-2467.

Plastic hula girls! Potato guns! Glow-in-the-dark cockroaches! Tiki God lamps! Revolving bow ties! Voodoo dolls! Squeaking rubber pickles! If all this makes no sense to you, just move on to the next entry, friend. But if you're tingling all over, fantasizing about how to make those glow-in-the-dark cockroaches into earrings, aching for a big boxful of useless plastic trinkets, you don't need us to tell you that you're a ready-made Archie McPhee customer. Archie McPhee has unarguably the best selection anywhere of tacky party favors, tasteless toys neglected in some warehouse since the 1950s, laughable religious souvenirs, JFK pencil sharpeners, and miniature plastic farm animals. Pointless to some, ambrosia to others. You know who you are.

Ashes in a Birdbath: in the Evergreen-Washelli Columbarium, Evergreen-Washelli Cemetery, east side of Aurora Avenue N, between N 110th Street and N 115th Street. Bus 6 goes right to the door. Open daily, 9 A.M.–5 P.M.

Not just any ashes, mind you: the burnt remains of a human body. To find the birdbath among the mazelike rows of urns, enter through the main door to the lobby, turn right, follow the row going left, then turn left at the next opportunity and look for a small birdbath with four white doves behind glass. If you get lost, which you will, ask an attendant to help you. She'll not only show you the birdbath but bring a stool for you to stand on and get a better view of the exposed ashes. While you're there, note some of the other unusual ash containers, like the mini-missile that contains an ex-Marine.

Bill Speidel's Underground Tour: tours start in Doc Maynard's Public House, 610 First Avenue, at Pioneer Square. Open March–September, daily; tours every hour on the hour, usually 11 A.M.–6 P.M. (10 A.M.–6 P.M. in July and August); hours vary slightly from month to month so call ahead to get tour times. Admission: $3.75; students, $3.25; seniors, $2.50; children 6–12, $2. Phone: For schedule, call (206) 682-1511; for reservations, call (206) 682-4646.

After a painfully honest lecture about the failures and foibles of Seattle's early history, sarcastic tour guides show you the part of town that never sees the light of day. Seattle was originally built too close to the tide level; after a disastrous fire in the late 1800s, the city was slowly rebuilt on a new, higher level. Large parts of the city were entombed as what was once the third story became the new ground level. The guides make plenty of plumbing and toilet jokes and are quick to point out idiotic and half-baked building schemes whose tacky underpinnings are plainly visible down here at foundation level. Only a small part of Seattle's eight-acre underground labyrinth is explored. "Underground Comedy Hour" might be a better name.

Campfire Museum: 8511 15th Avenue NE, northeast of Green Lake. Open by appointment only. Admission: free. Phone: (206) 524-8550.

Wood Gatherers and Path Finders of every vintage will get a funny, warm feeling inside, looking over this Campfire memorabilia, much of which was donated by octogenarian Campfire Girls. On display are ceremonial gowns, bead-studded vests, scrapbooks, Blue Bird costumes (don't *ever* call them uniforms, young lady), and an exhibit of Campfire candy (sales of which, interestingly, were preceded by sales of Campfire *donuts*). The old Camp Sealth photos from the 1930s and 1940s show bobbed hair, handsome horses, and happy girls. Note to former Campfire Girls: Wo He Lo.

Dancing Bronze Footprints: along both sides of Broadway from E Denny Way to E Roy Street. Always visible.

Some days, you're swinging down the street, snapping your fingers, head in the clouds, worries a million miles away, and you feel like dancing! But—oh no! What if you don't know the steps? Not to worry, if the street you're on is Broadway, because on Broadway the sidewalk itself teaches you how to dance, using the tried-and-true numbered-footsteps-and-arrows technique. Here are the dances and their locations: (1) The Bus Stop: southwest corner of Broadway and Denny Way. (2) The Tango: northeast corner of Broadway and Denny Way. (3) The Waltz: southwest corner of Broadway and Olive Way. (4) The Rumba: east side of Broadway between John Way and Thomas Way. (5) The Mambo: west side of Broadway between Thomas Way and Harrison Way. (6) Foxtrot Weave: southeast corner of Broadway and Republican Way. (7) Obeebo: northwest corner of Broadway and Republican Way. (8) The Lindy: southwest corner of Broadway and Roy Street.

Gas Works Park Human Sundial: in Gas Works Park, on N Northlake Way, on the promontory sticking out into the northern end of Lake Union; sundial is on top of the park's hill. From downtown, take bus 26 north and walk from N 35th Street and Wallingford Avenue N. Always visible. Admission: free. Phone: (206) 625-4223.

Rain-soaked Seattle isn't the greatest place for a sundial. This one, however, is interesting in any weather, and it works as a moondial, too. *You* become part of the sundial: it's your shadow that points to what time it is. Stand on one of the 12 little suns (according to what month it is), face your shadow, and...Oh, my God, it's 3:30! I had an appointment at 3:00! Inlaid into the multicolored cement sundial are shards of porcelain, glass, beads, and shells. Art nouveau numbers and astrological figures tell you the time and the sign.

Goodwill "Memory Lane" Museum: 1400 S Lane Street (at Dearborn), south of downtown. (From downtown, take bus 26 south.) Museum is at the rear of the store. Open Monday–Friday, 10 A.M.–6 P.M.; Saturday, 9 A.M.–5 P.M.; Sunday, 10 A.M.–5 P.M. Admission: free. Phone: (206) 329-1000.

For 20 years, Seattle's Goodwill—probably the world's largest thrift store—has been saving its best donations and putting them on display in this museum. We're talking prime-choice castoffs, the kind of stuff you wish you could have discovered yourself and taken home for $1.95: Victorian gowns, political buttons, totem poles, mandolins, kiddie tea sets...and every bit of it culled from donation bins. Most exhibits have a historical theme: the "Flapper's Bedroom" has art deco pottery, jazzy sheet music, and a boffo pair of shoes.

Highline School District Museum: 15631 8th Avenue S at SW 156th Street, in the Sunnydale district. Open Thursday, 10 A.M.–noon and 1–4 P.M., and the second and fourth Saturdays of every month from September to June, 10 A.M.–noon and 1–4 P.M. Also open by appointment. Admission: free. Phone: (206) 433-2391 or (206) 433-2447.

Housed in a defunct elementary school, the museum has life-size dioramas that show what school was like in the days of long division and apples for the teacher. In one classroom, a stern but kindly schoolmarm mannequin doles out the three Rs and the values of middle-class society, ready to smack any student who talks back. Another room shows the principal's tiny office, and another is a replica of the first school in the area—which was in the teacher's kitchen.

Jimi Hendrix Memorial: in the Woodland Park Zoo, South Gate entrance at N 50th Street and Fremont Avenue N. Open daily, 8:30 A.M.–dusk. Admission: $3; seniors and children 6–17, $1.50; children under 6, free. Phone: (206) 789-7919.

Enter the south gate; walk straight ahead past the snack booth. Turn right and go about 200 feet until you see a sign that reads "Savannah Safari Continues"; turn left into the Savannah Overlook, next to the Savannah Birdhouse. On a large undulating rock you'll see a sun-shaped bronze marker, dedicating this Savannah Viewpoint to the "memory of Jimi Hendrix and his music." Jimi was a native of Seattle. But why oh why is the city's sole memorial to him inside the *zoo?* The zoo's more accessible and more interesting than Jimi's actual grave (south of Seattle, in Renton). But still.... This memorial is odder than it is thrilling; but for Hendrixheads who just have to "stand next to his fire"—this is it.

Lutefisk Eating Contest: last Saturday in July, around noon. Bergen Place Park, corner of 22nd Avenue NW and NW Market Street, in the Ballard suburb, west of Green Lake. For more information, call (206) 783-0535.

Lutefisk, a Scandinavian delicacy, is cod prepared with lye. *Lye.* Lutefisk looks like lumpy Cream of Wheat and smells...well, you can imagine. To pronounce it like a proper Viking, you must use three syllables: *loo-ta-fisk.* To eat it, you must be crazy, or else a hardcore Norwegian. A recent contest winner managed to bolt down eight pounds of the stuff in the two minutes allotted to him. Yikes.

Marzi Tarts Erotic Bakery: 2323 N 45th Street (at Sunnyside). Take bus 26 from downtown. Open Tuesday–Saturday, 10:30 A.M.–6:30 P.M.; Monday, 11 A.M.–6 P.M. Phone: (206) 328-2253 (EAT-CAKE).

Marzi Tarts' cupcakes are more than just edible. They're exact replicas of perky body parts that we won't mention here because our editor won't let us. You should *see* what these folks can do with marzipan! Leaf through the shop's mouth-watering, spine-tingling catalog of made-to-order cakes, and you'll see cakes shaped like things, cakes with things sticking out of them, cakes with things sticking into them....

"Melting Ice" Building: on the 700 block of Roy Street, next to Queen Anne Avenue N. Always visible.

Silent, abandoned, and lacking an address, this strange bit of architecture looks like a pile of melting ice, a well-toasted marshmallow without the black crust, or perhaps the cake that was left out in the rain in MacArthur Park. The "roof" is a series of asymmetrical, undulating white humps; the overall shape defies all architectural and aesthetic sensibilities. Its function and history are lost in the mists of time, its future the greatest mystery of all.

Milk Carton Derby: during the early part of Seafair, usually on a weekend in mid-July. At the boating area on the southern end of Green Lake, off Green Lake Drive N in north central Seattle. Race is from 10 A.M.–3 P.M. For current date and more information, call (206) 623-7100.

What are empty milk cartons good for, besides identifying runaway children and taking up too much space in the kitchen garbage can? Hell, it's obvious, ain't it? You make *boats* out of 'em: boats shaped like hippopotami and elephants; boats shaped like airplanes, trucks, and dragons; boats shaped like 900 smelly milk cartons glued haphazardly together. Then you climb on board and paddle around Green Lake in front of thousands of jeering Seattleites.

Royal Brougham Sports Museum: inside the Kingdome, 201 S King Street. Open during the hours just before (and sometimes after) a sporting event in the Kingdome, and at the end of tours of the Kingdome (April–September, Monday–Saturday, 11 A.M., 1 and 3 P.M., starting at Gate D. Tours cost $2.50; children, $1.25). Admission: free, but you have to pay to get into the sporting event or to go on the tour. Phone: (206) 340-2128. Call to confirm times.

No, Royal Brougham is not Queen Elizabeth's carriage. He was the sports editor of the Seattle *Post-Intelligencer*. During his long career, Brougham collected sports memorabilia. His collection formed the nucleus of the museum that now bears his name. A high point here is a pair of boxing shorts signed by Muhammad Ali. And don't miss Pelé's soccer jersey. Also here are press passes from memorable sports events and other clothing and knickknacks of the stars.

Sand Castle Contest: usually the second Sunday in August, but times may be changed because of Seafair events. Contest starts at 9 A.M.; judging is around 3:30 P.M. On Alki Beach, southwest Seattle. For exact date and more information, call (206) 684-7430.

This big-city sand castle competition, called Sandblast, draws upward of 4,000 spectators. Big cash prizes, various categories in which to compete, and plenty of publicity make this another key event in the sand castle circuit.

Sound Garden and Moby Dick Bridges: on the grounds of the National Oceanic and Atmospheric Administration (NOAA) headquarters, 7600 Sand Point Way NE, north of Magnuson Park on Lake Washington. If you enter from Sand Point Way, keep to the left (north) of the buildings and follow the waterfront path all the way to the other side of the buildings. If you enter from Magnuson Park, the only gate through the fence is right at the water's edge, and the path leads directly from the gate to the bridge and sound garden. Buses 74, 75, and 41 go right to the main entrance. Open daily, daylight hours. Admission: free. For more information, call the Seattle Arts Commission: (206) 625-4223.

You may want to ask, "Why do these two identical bridges span dry land? Why are they both covered with the exact same quotes from *Moby Dick*, set in bronze letters?" But don't say it out loud. Your only answer will be a faint moan from the Sound Garden, which is a sophisticated wind organ: one dozen 20-foot pipes controlled by rudders and rotating in the wind. Air passing through slots in the pipes creates dissonant toots and howls, giving you the feeling that this is the last day on Earth before the aliens arrive. "Then all collapsed and the great shroud of the sea rolled on as it rolled 5000 years ago." Don't ask.

Statue of Liberty Replica: near Alki Beach, next to the intersection of Alki Avenue SW and 63rd Avenue SW. Always visible. Admission: free. For more information, call (206) 684-7430.

"I know they moved London Bridge to Arizona, but when did they move the Statue of Liberty out here?" This eight-foot exact replica of the Statue of Liberty has had plenty of confused foreign tourists wondering what coast they're on. "It looks so much bigger on the TV." The statue, facing out to sea on a tall pedestal, is entitled "The Birthplace of Seattle Monument" and is supposed to commemorate Seattle's founding. Why they felt compelled to reuse someone else's statue is beyond us.

Waterfall Garden: northwest corner of Main Street and 2nd Avenue S. Open daily, 10 A.M.–8 P.M. Admission: free. For more information, call (206) 447-4200.

Twenty-five feet of water surge and crash mightily, a scant few yards from bustling downtown traffic. Built in honor of the men and women of the United Parcel Service, this artificial waterfall makes a dramatically loud noise and lots of refreshing mist. Urbanites snack and kibbitz all around it, and exuberant ferns complete the sylvan-urban scene.

Ye Olde Curiosity Shop: Pier 54, Alaskan Way, on the waterfront just south of Pike Place Market. Open daily, 9 A.M.–9 P.M. Admission: free. Phone: (206) 682-5844.

Your Seattle friends might refuse to take you to see this 90-year-old curio emporium, denouncing it as "too famous." Sure, it's famous, but you *must* see it because it has on display the Lord's Prayer on a grain of rice; two 19th-century human mummies; a stillborn fawn in a jar; the world's smallest shrunken head; a mummified dog; a headless seal; a tugboat made of matchsticks; a mummified rat; Mount Rushmore on a grain of rice; a shrunken Jivaro Indian torso; totem poles; the world's smallest safety pin; a chain carved from a single toothpick; a whale's eardrum; a piglet with two heads, three eyes, and eight legs; a 67-pound snail; the smallest coins ever minted; a quarter-inch silver spoon; fleas wearing dresses; and a duckbill platypus.

SPOKANE

The Crosby Library: East 502 Boone Avenue, just behind the Administration Building at Gonzaga University. Open Monday–Friday, 8 A.M.–10 P.M.; Saturday 9 A.M.–1 P.M.; Sunday, 4–8 P.M. Admission: free. Phone: (509) 328-4220, ext. 3132.

The crooner's gold records, photos, and personal artifacts line all four walls of this library/shrine. Over 20 gold records are in the collection, as are several of Bing's Oscars. Gonzaga was Crosby's alma mater.

STEVENSON

(On the Columbia River)

World's Largest Rosary Collection: in the Skamania County Museum, basement of the Courthouse Annex, Vancouver Avenue between Columbia and Russell Streets. Open Monday–Saturday, noon–5 P.M.; Sunday, 1–6 P.M. Admission: free. Phone: (509) 427-5141, ext. 235.

A rosary made of bullets, a glow-in-the-dark rosary, the JFK WWII rosary...these are just a sampling of the nearly 4,000 specimens in this startling collection. A local man spent his entire life collecting rosaries, then donated them to this museum. Today they occupy a whole room, kept company by plaster statues of saints. The rosaries come from all over the world. Some are unbelievably tiny, and the largest is ten feet long, with "beads" made of fishing floats.

TACOMA

Bed Race: second Saturday in August. Parade begins 11
A.M.; race begins noon; Pacific Avenue between 9th and
13th. For more information, call (206) 572-4200.

If you're into those high-speed, wham-bam-thank-ya-
ma'am soulless bed races, then you've come to the wrong
place. Tacoma's bed race aims for laughs, as participants
dress in their funniest pajamas. Beds, too, are dressed according to a variety of themes.

Bing Crosby Historical Society: 902 Commerce Street
(at 9th), in the Pantages Center. Open Monday–Friday,
11 A.M.–3 P.M., and by appointment. Admission: free.
Phone: (206) 627-2947.

"The fella that was born to sing, the fella that the
world called Bing....Others have come, others have gone;
none was as great; none lasted as long." That's the cheery
brand of fandom you'll find around here, summed up in a
framed poem that hangs on the wall. Also here are a Bing
Crosby clock and pictures of Bing playing a ukulele,
wearing a coolie hat, and standing around limp-wristedly.
One incongruous artifact is a life-size ceramic dog with a
choke chain. The placard reads, "Ping—donated by a
blind member from Akron, Ohio."

Java Jive: 2102 South Tacoma Way, at Ferry Street
next to Interstate 5, southwest of downtown. Open Monday–Thursday, 3 P.M.–midnight; Friday, 3 P.M.–2 A.M.;
Saturday, 6 P.M.–2 A.M. Closed Sunday. Admission: free.
Phone: (206) 475-9843.

Tacoma is the only place where you can get your coffee

out of a coffee pot *in* a coffee pot.
Confused? Java Jive is a coffee-pot-
shaped restaurant and lounge.
Built in 1927, it's still in excellent
condition, white with a ruddy-
brown spout, handle, and lid. The
inside has a jungle/driftwood/ 1960s kitsch theme, replete
with spray-painted game trophies, African masks, and
fishing floats. Bathrooms are labeled "Tarzan" and
"Jane." (The owner used to keep live apes on the
premises, too, but no longer.) The Java Jive's many wild
incarnations—as speakeasy, go-go dance club, and home
base for the Ventures—mingle and permeate the atmosphere.

Never Never Land: in Point Defiance Park, far northern tip of the city. Open June–Labor Day, daily, 10 A.M.–7 P.M.; April–May, daily, 10 A.M.–5 P.M. March, Saturday and Sunday only, 10 A.M.–5 P.M. Admission: $1.50; children 13–17, $1.25; children 3–12, 75¢; children under 3, free. Phone: (206) 591-5845.

If fairies really do exist, then this is where they live: in this European-style storybook forest. Dozens of artfully crafted, lovingly detailed scenes nestle amid tall, cool hemlocks. They really, really don't make 'em like this anymore. Each scene keeps you standing and staring forever: polka-dot-clad kittens scrub their mittens with grim determination; Simple Simon's pieman beams with pride at his wares. Note the giant bookcase that serves as gateway to Never Never Land, and be sure to pose for a picture inside Peter's enormous pumpkin.

TENINO
(15 miles south of Olympia)

Wolf Haven: 3111 Offut Lake Road, three miles north of town. From Highway 5, take exit 99 to 93rd Street. Follow this to the intersection of old Highway 99. Turn right on 99 and go three miles. Open for tours in summer, daily, 10 A.M.–5 P.M. (Tour hours reduced in winter.) Howl-ins: summer only, Friday and Saturday, 7–10 P.M. Admission to tours: $3; children 6–15, $2; children under 6, free. Howl-ins: $4; children 6–15, $2.50; children under 6, free. Phone: (206) 264-HOWL or (800) 448-WOLF.

Who's afraid of the big bad wolf? Too many people, and for all the wrong reasons, says the group that runs this 60-acre wolf sanctuary. They're determined to teach you what wolves are really like. Myths are dispelled with wild abandon as you meet several dozen real live wolves—each with a name and personality all its own. At the evening Howl-ins, staff and storytellers share with visitors the beauty of wolves in folklore and song, as you toast marshmallows and yell, "Awoo!"

TOUTLE
(25 miles northeast of Kelso)

Mount St. Helens Museum: in the North Toutle 19 Mile House, which is 19 miles east of Highway 5 on

Highway 504. Official address is 9440 Spirit Lake Highway. Open daily, 8 A.M.–8 P.M. Admission: $1. Phone: (206) 274-8779.

Want to relive those glorious days of May 1980, when Mount St. Helens flattened forests, melted cars, obliterated rivers, and blackened the skies? Displays at this museum tell the Mount St. Helens story before, during, and after the eruption—but especially *during*. You know, the good part: eighty jillion cubic miles of ash in the air; avalanches of mud wiping out entire species; trees scattered like toothpicks. America is still number one! We even have the best volcanoes!

UNION
(30 miles northwest of Olympia)

Seagull Calling Contest: the Saturday preceding Memorial Day, 11 A.M.–1 P.M. Alderbrook Resort, East 7101 Highway 106 (106 is the main road through town). For more information, call (206) 898-4351.

Contestants coax gulls right out of the sky and onto a 10-by-20-foot landing zone. They do this by screeching, keening, hopping on one foot, and flapping their arms. The weird thing is, it works. Last year's winner managed to summon nine gullible gulls. For $2 you can have your chance to play St. Francis, but remember what the locals say: There's a fine line between attracting gulls and scaring them away.

VANTAGE
(28 miles east of Ellensburg)

Ginkgo Petrified Forest State Park: three miles west of Vantage on the Vantage Highway, which runs parallel to and one mile north of Highway 90. Open in summer, 6:30 A.M.–dusk, in winter, 8 A.M.–5 P.M. Admission: free. Phone: (509) 856-2700.

Long ago, when most of Washington was a big swamp, oceans of lava came out of nowhere and inundated the whole area. The lava hardened and became rock. Over the ensuing millennia, the rock eroded to reveal that ancient water-soaked logs at the bottom of the swamp had been preserved by the lava rather than incinerated by it. The logs were petrified. Some of these logs were ginkgo trees, a rare species that no longer exists in the wild—only in nurseries. The ones here are the only examples of petrified ginkgo anywhere in the world. A three-quarter-mile trail leads through the petrified forest. The interpretive center, 2½ miles east, has explanatory exhibits, polished petrified wood, and even live ginkgo trees.

WALLA WALLA

Renaissance Faire: last Saturday in April, 10 A.M.–3 P.M. Activities are centered around the Memorial Building, Whitman College Campus, Boyer Avenue at Park Street. Admission: free. For more information, call (509) 527-5169.

Jugglers, fencers, and Renaissance dance troupes hold workshops so that faire-goers might, prithee, get themselves ye olde education. Also on campus for the event is a real Shakespearean actor, whose rousing renditions of the Bard's works involve audience participation. Renaissance-type food and crafts booths, jousters, and fortune tellers round out the jollity.

Sweet Onion Festival: fourth Sunday in July, noon–5 P.M. Fort Walla Walla Museum Complex, Myra Road (at Rose). Admission: $1. Phone: (509) 383-2223 or (509) 525-0850.

Not a single tear falls at the onion slicing contest. That's because these onions are sweet: Walla Wallans say you can chomp 'em like apples. The festival features an onion recipe contest (onion ice cream is not unheard of around here), onion decorating contest, onion slicing contest (based on thinness of slice), and an onion hunt. A recent champion of the double-headed onion shot put hurled his mutated vegetable 85 feet, and ended up in the *Guinness Book of World Records*. The season's largest onion wins a prize, too: Last year's measured nearly 20 inches around.

WESTPORT

Fleet Blessing: the Sunday preceding Memorial Day, usually around noon. At the extreme tip of the peninsula, near the Fishermen's Memorial. For more information, call (206) 268-9422 or (800) 345-6223.

Hey, Jack, that's no kiddie pool out there. It's the open ocean, and many a member of the local tuna- and salmon-fishing fleet has been lost at sea. Westport remembers the lost ones and blesses the living ones at this event, with songs and a procession. The Coast Guard, flying overhead in a helicopter, drops a wreath into the foaming sea.

WOODINVILLE
(15 miles northeast of Seattle)

All Fools' Day Parade and Basset Bash: the Saturday nearest April 1. Parade begins 1 P.M.; goes down Northeast 175th Street. Basset Bash also begins 1 P.M., in the schoolyard, 13209 Northeast 175th Street. For more information, call (206) 483-0606.

The Basset Bash is a heck of a beauty contest. Sad-eyed bowsers from four states are judged on length of ears, soulfulness of howl, and other pertinent criteria. Participants receive "Bona Phideaux" certificates, and winners receive basset pizzas—made of ground-up dog biscuits and baked in the shape of dog biscuits. Meanwhile, the All Fools' Parade attracts the kind of fools we like: Last year, a man arrived dressed as a shower, complete with sprinklers. One of the "floats" was a wagon bearing a dead halibut. Rose Parade, hit the high road.

ZILLAH
(20 miles southeast of Yakima)

Teapot Dome Service Station: Take exit 54 off Highway 82 coming southeast from Yakima; you can see it just before you exit, on the right (southwest) side of the road. Open daily, 6 A.M.–6 P.M., but visible anytime. Phone: (509) 829-6994.

Awww, ain't this the cutest little gas station you ever saw? This single-room, red and white teapot has the most delicate and finely crafted handle and spout of any of the teapot-shaped edifices we've come across. The teapot, of course, isn't the whole station—just the office. The pumps are out front.

NEVADA

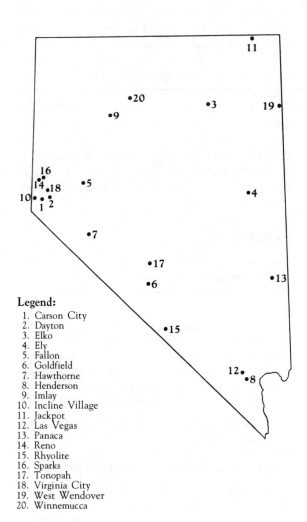

Legend:
1. Carson City
2. Dayton
3. Elko
4. Ely
5. Fallon
6. Goldfield
7. Hawthorne
8. Henderson
9. Imlay
10. Incline Village
11. Jackpot
12. Las Vegas
13. Panaca
14. Reno
15. Rhyolite
16. Sparks
17. Tonopah
18. Virginia City
19. West Wendover
20. Winnemucca

Only a few select states have their own special themes: Hawaii's got surfing, Utah's got Mormons, and New Jersey's got pollution. Nevada once achieved notoriety as the country's only remaining frontier state, but the real Wild West slipped away into the history books shortly after *The Misfits* was filmed here. With the rise of the Las Vegas ethic, Nevada embraced a new state theme, one that had actually been there all along: gambling. Nevadans have always gambled—hell, in the old days even coming to Nevada was a gamble. Risk-takers and speculators were drawn to this wide-open state, looking to strike it rich mining silver or robbing stagecoaches. The few that did make money squandered it on fantan and bear fights. It didn't take long for locals to realize that the real way to rake in the cash was to run a casino. It's been uphill since then. Now tourists the world over flock to Nevada for the sole purpose of gambling away their money. As the state's economy prospers, the Nevadans grin slyly; this is a lot easier than rustling cattle.

CARSON CITY

Gold Nugget Collection: in the entrance to the Carson Nugget Casino, 507 North Carson Street. Open daily, 24 hours. Admission: free. Phone: (702) 882-1626.

It gives us the shivers to look at all those rows of nuggets—not just because of their combined value, which is about a million dollars, but also because of the beauty of the gold itself. In its natural state, the stuff is raw and luminous. In the collection are weirdly shaped examples of leaf gold, thread gold, ribbon gold, and wire gold; gold flakes; gold chunks; gold globules. Sorry, no free samples.

Kit Carson Rendezvous: second week in June. Mills Park, east of downtown, three blocks blocks off Highway 50E. Wagon train arrives at the rendezvous 10 A.M. Saturday. Phone: (800) 634-8700 or (702) 883-7442.

A whoopin' wagon train, having rolled all the way across the valley from Reno, roars into Carson City Saturday morning. Buckskin-clad mountain men and Indians join the dusty wagoneers in a peace-pipe ceremony, kicking off the rendezvous. One section of the park is transformed into the Indian Village, where Nevada tribes occupy tents and tipis, dance, and serve Indian tacos. Elsewhere in the park is the Mountain Men's Encampment; rugged guys in fringed costumes recall the days of the fur trade. At the Ferriers' Contest, folks pound horseshoes out of raw metal chunks; and down by the creek, cannons flare as "soldiers" reenact a Civil War battle.

Nevada Day Celebration: October 31. Bed race: 9:30 A.M., down North Carson Street in front of the State Library. Rock-drilling contest: 11 A.M. in the Nugget parking lot, 507 North Carson Street. Beard contest judging: 1:30 P.M., in front of the State Capitol, Carson Street (at King). For more information, call (800) 634-8700 or (702) 882-1565.

They celebrate the state's birthday this way, with competitions in two of Nevada's oldest traditions: mining and beard growing. Rock drillers get ten minutes to see how deeply they can penetrate a hunk of solid granite, using an old-time single-jack drill. (Some recent winners drilled 12 inches.) Beards are judged in various categories: blackest, reddest, longest, etc. The bed race is a high-speed, high-pressure event.

Nevada State Prison Hobby Store: corner of East 5th Street and Edmonds, far eastern end of town, near the foothills. Open daily, 6:30 A.M.–4:30 P.M. Admission: free. Phone: (702) 887-3285.

Engaged? Planning to put your name on the bridal registry at Macy's? Why not try something different this time around: Register at the Prison Hobby Store. They sell wallets, belt buckles, stuffed animals, yarn art, scarves—everything you'll need to start a new life together. This is definitely the most unusual crafts shop in Nevada. Artistic prisoners sell their creations here, and the selection is always changing. Keep those inmates in pocket money as they hone their skills making fake weapons for the big breakout.

Whistle-Off: third weekend in August. Mills Park, east of downtown, three blocks off Highway 50E. Events are concentrated in the far left end of the park. For more information, call (800) 634-8700 or (702) 882-1565.

Serious twitterers from all over the globe wrap their lips around classical melodies, popular tunes, and novelty numbers. This last category is the wackiest of all, as contestants are permitted to incorporate comedy, costumes, and really bizarre melodies. Hearing these virtuoso puckerers perform Beethoven makes you realize, if you hadn't already, that the human head is an instrument in its own right.

DAYTON
(Ten miles east of Carson City)

Bed Race: the Saturday closest to August 16. Procession begins at 2 P.M., St. Anne's Mission Church, Pike Street. Bed race follows procession. For more information, call (702) 246-3435.

Who *says* you can't celebrate the Assumption of Mary with a bed race? A procession of young girls ("They're supposed to be virgins," a Dayton local informs us) accompanies the priest and a statue of Mary down the street in an attitude of piety. Then the statue leads the racing beds (and other things, admittedly) in a parade. Finally, the beds elbow out the competition and race wildly down Pike Street.

ELKO

Cowboy Poetry Gathering: the last weekend in January (Thursday–Saturday). Elko Convention Center, Cedar Street at Festival Way, downtown. Admission to poetry readings: free. Cowboy music events have variable fees. A festival badge ($5) gets you into all nonfree events. For more information, call (702) 738-7508.

Cowboy poetry—blazingly real tales of the real West, by people who know—has been around for a long time, but only recently have tenderfeet become privy to it. It's catching on like—well, like wildfire, podner. At the festival, real cowboys and cowgirls recite works on such themes as "Good Rides and Bad Horses," "Women on the Ranch," and "Cowboy Heroes." By night, guitars cry and boot heels tap to the tune of cowboy classics. We're talkin' "Lone Prairie" here, not "Rhinestone Cowboy."

Man-Mule Race: first Saturday in October. All day. Route varies from year to year, but always includes the towns of Elko and Lamoille (20 miles south of Elko). For current route and other information, call (702) 738-7135.

Men and mules battle it out to see who's fastest. But whereas the mules have only their legs to rely on, the wily humans use bicycles, skis, roller skates, and even more unconventional conveyances, thus increasing their own odds considerably. As long as it's nonmotorized, it's fair game. Man and beast toil all day along the 18-to-20-mile course, while bystanders cheer and bray.

FALLON

Musical Sand Dune: at Sand Mountain, 24 miles southeast of Fallon, just north of Highway 50. Look for a large, white, smooth mountain on the edge of a dry lakebed; it is visible from the highway, and there is a turnoff. For more information, call the Fallon Naval Air Station at (702) 426-2716.

This desert dune, also known as the Singing Mountain, has the eerie habit of making sounds of its own accord. Something about the size, shape, and composition of the grains makes them hum, rumble, and growl as they vibrate and rub against each other. Optimum time to visit is when it's hot, arid, and windy. Luckily, in this hellish desert it's almost always hot, arid, and windy. The tough part, however, is finding a day on which there are no big-wheeled motorcycles and dune buggies roaring up and down the mountain. The "singing" sands are too delicate to compete with the internal combustion engine.

GOLDFIELD

Treasure Days: second weekend in August. World barstool sitting championship: 6 P.M. Saturday, Goldfield Hotel, Highway 95. Greased pig tussle: 3 P.M. Saturday and Sunday, old ballpark, Main Street. Miners' Liars' contest: 11 A.M. Sunday, Goldfield Hotel. For more information, call (702) 485-6365.

Barstool sitting is much more difficult than falling off a log. Judging is based on technique of approach, mounting, and actual sitting. Past contestants have drunk beer out of boots, let off helium balloons, and cried. A recent winner was a beer-swilling, 450-pound sow that sings. All the fibs in the Miners' Liars' contest must be mining-related, which is only appropriate in this former gold-rush town. Kids tackle greased pigs and a greased pole. They also force costumed horned toads to race each other, and they play on a miniature golf course whose last "hole" is an outhouse. Finally, the Cactus Cookoff produces candy, stew, chili—you'd be amazed at what you can make with cactus, once you figure out what to do with the spines.

HAWTHORNE

Cecil the Sea Serpent: on display in the public works storage yard on O Street at 10th Street. Always open, but visible only from behind a chain-link fence. For more information, call (702) 945-5896.

In Walker Lake, north of Hawthorne, dwells a terrifying monster, surrounded by legends. The local Indians called him Toagwa. When Mineral County adopted the monster as its mascot, white folks had a hard time pronouncing Toagwa, so they changed the name to Cecil. In 1964 they built a 100-foot Cecil float for the Nevada centennial parade, and they've hauled it out for special occasions ever since. Between special occasions, you can see Cecil in a storage yard. The float has a huge head and gaping mouth, a howdah perched on one of its humps, and sharklike fins. Plans are underway to move Cecil to a new location, so if he's not in the storage yard when you visit, ask for directions to his new home.

Liars' Race: third Sunday in June; first race at 9 A.M.; main race at noon. On Walker Lake, at the boating area off Highway 95, about 12 miles north of town. For more information, call (702) 945-5896.

This race has nothing to do with telling lies or going fast. It has to do with building the craziest boat your imagination will allow and puttering around on the lake very slowly. Every year the regatta gets funnier; some of the crafts wreak havoc on the very definition of "boat." The only requirement is that the vehicles stay afloat. Spectators are welcomed.

HENDERSON

Ethel M Chocolate Factory and Cactus Garden: 2 Cactus Garden Drive, west of Highway 95 (Boulder Highway), near the intersection of Mountain Vista Street and Sunset Road, just southeast of downtown Las Vegas. Open daily, 9 A.M.–5:30 P.M. Admission: free. Phone: (702) 458-8864.

Ham and eggs, chicken and dumplings, liver and onions, and...chocolate and cactus? Nobody does chocolate and cactus like Ethel M. Okay, you aren't expected to eat the cactus, but I don't like liver either, so we're even. A brief narrated tour of this homey gourmet candy factory (whose specialty is liqueur chocolates) climaxes with a free sample. Eat this before venturing out into the cactus garden, for the desert heat shows no mercy on chocolates. The garden is impressive and flawless, with ocotillo, Clokey's cholla, aloe vera, prickly pear, and 350 other spiny specimens. A sign warns, "Please be careful. Cactus bite."

IMLAY
(40 miles northeast of Lovelock)

Chief Rolling Mountain Thunder's Monument: on the frontage road just off Interstate 80, just up from the sheriff substation. Stay outside the fence unless invited in. For more information, call the Nevada Arts Council at (702) 789-0225.

The chief's eccentric, exuberant, and angry personal vision takes shape in burgeoning cement warrens, studded with what some might call debris: old cans, bits of bicycles, car parts, bones, beads, glass.... Locals—even locals in the art community—call the chief's work "trash statuary." All over the property are sculptures, statues, stacks of cars, and venomous signs protesting the Bureau of Land Management's mustang-control policy. You might even see a dead horse propped up against a hand-painted "Indian curse" against the BLM. Remember, when you visit, that this is private property.

INCLINE VILLAGE

Ponderosa Ranch: 1½ miles southeast of town on Highway 28, on the east side of the road. Follow the signs. Open May–October, daily, 10 A.M.–5 P.M.; hours are extended to 10 A.M.–6 P.M. around midsummer. Admission: $5.50; children 5–11, $4.50; children under 5, free. Phone: (702) 831-0691.

"We got a right to pick a little fight—BONANZA!" It used to be a TV show; now it's a theme park. In the show, the Ponderosa Ranch was south of Virginia City, near Lake Tahoe. This set, where the show was filmed, is south of Virginia City, near Lake Tahoe. "Bonanza" was actually filmed where it was supposed to be taking place! Relive the wasted hours you spent sitting in front of the TV by chowing down on Hossburgers as stuntmen "die" in mock gunfights. Also here are the Mystery Mine (balls rolling uphill, etc.), a petting farm, a mock western town, the real Ponderosa ranch house, and more. "If anyone fights any one of us, he's gotta fight with me!"

JACKPOT
(68 miles north of Wells)

Hollering Contest: July 4, 2 P.M. Shoshone Canyon, one-half mile south of town. From Jackpot, go south one-quarter mile on New Highway 93. Turn right through a barbed-wire gate and go 500 yards to the west, where you'll come to Old Highway 93. Turn left there and enter the canyon. Warning: Old 93 is a rough road. Parking and turning cars around in the canyon are difficult, and there are no toilets. For more information, call (702) 755-2259.

When Nevada pioneers of yore wanted to get messages to their neighbors, they "gave a holler"—literally. A long, wavering yell could fill a whole valley and was as good as Morse code for getting the idea across: "My wife just had a baby." "Anyone need anything from town?" The hollering contest revives this pretelephone skill. Entrants in pioneer costume are judged on the basis of pitch, sound, and length of holler.

LAS VEGAS

The American Museum of Historical Documents: 3200 South Las Vegas Boulevard, lower level of the Fashion Show Mall. Open Monday–Wednesday, 10 A.M.–6 P.M.; Thursday–Friday, 10 A.M.–9 P.M.; Sunday, noon–5 P.M. Closed Saturday. Admission: free. Phone: (702) 731-0785.

Next time you win $34,990 on one pull of a nickel slot machine, take the cash straight over to this museum/gallery and plonk it down on a letter signed by John F. Kennedy. According to the museum's director, you couldn't make a better investment. He's made a bundle in the document business himself. The range of letters, cards, proclamations, and notes on display here, signed by famous people, is amazing—and most of them are for sale: Ingrid Bergman, George Washington, Wyatt Earp, Albert Einstein, Bruce Lee, Sitting Bull, Walt Disney, and more.

Brahma Shrine: in front of Caesar's Palace, 3570 Las Vegas Boulevard South, to the right of the main fountain as you enter from the street, near the covered walkway. Always open. Admission: free. Phone: (702) 731-7110.

This is no gimmick to amuse passersby. It's a real shrine. People actually worship here. They leave offerings of fruit, flowers, and plastic leis. A bronze statue of Brahma with four beneficent faces sits in the center, gazing mildly in all directions, surrounded by hundreds of carved elephants. Most of the worshippers are Asian and Indian tourists, shoring up their credit with the Big One upstairs before venturing into the casino. But often as not you'll find a WASP with a "Why not?" expression kneeling and praying, too.

Caesar's World: in front of Caesar's Palace, 3570 Las Vegas Boulevard South, to the right of the main fountain as you face the casino, at the entrance to the covered walkway. Always open. Admission: free. Phone: (702) 731-7110.

A real live Roman Centurion, shield and all, greets you at the entrance to the simulated Roman temple. Enter the dark doorway and a moving walkway whisks you into ten seconds of Roman fantasy, à la hologram. Roman feasts and orgies shimmer on either side of you. Suddenly, little hologram people run screaming from a burning villa. It's over before you know it, and it's hard to catch all the action the first time through. So go back for another ride.

Coca-Cola Museum: in Calamity Jane's Ice Cream House, which is in Sam's Town Casino, east of downtown at 5111 Boulder Highway (at Nellis). Open daily, 9 A.M.–11 P.M. Admission: free. Phone: (702) 456-7777.

All that's missing is the fizz and the cocaine. Coca-Cola artifacts fill nearly every inch of wall space in this ice-cream parlor. A giant Coke bottle, over three feet tall, looms like a caffeinated nightmare behind glass; other giant bottles stand against walls and bay windows. A framed case holds a century's worth of Coca-Cola pins; elsewhere you can inspect antique signs, calendars, souvenirs, and bottles, bottles, bottles.

Liberace Museum: 1775 East Tropicana. Open Monday–Saturday, 10 A.M.–5 P.M.; Sunday, 1–5 P.M. Admission: $6.50; seniors, $4.50; children under 12, $2. Phone: (702) 798-5595.

So it's a museum dedicated to excessive extravagance, glitz, and flamboyance. Are you surprised? One building (the museum consists of three separate, distinct areas) is full of Liberace's pianos and cars, all in sparkling condition and each with some extraordinary history. Another section houses "the million-dollar wardrobe," with racks and racks of mahvelous capes, furs, and other clothes. The Liberace Library has scrapbooks, articles, gold and platinum records, and piano-shaped music boxes. To cap off your visit to the headquarters of Liberace worship, follow the Liberace timeline plaques to the Liberace gift shop.

Lucky Forest: in Fitzgerald's Casino, 301 East Fremont Street (at Third), downtown. Lucky Forest is on the main floor. Open daily, 8 A.M.–10 P.M. Admission: free. Phone: (702) 388-2400. No one under 21 is allowed in the casino.

If you think finding a single four-leaf clover is lucky, how'd you like to soak up the luck cascading from a crystal ball containing 10,000 four-leaf clovers? Also in this luck museum is the ultimate lucky horseshoe—it was worn by Secretariat, the winningest horse in history. Other exhibits explore symbols of good and bad luck, both familiar and obscure: two-tailed lizards and medicine bags, for example. Ascend the Wishing Steps made of "Blarney stones" (taken from Ireland's Blarney Castle) to the Echoing Wishing Well. (The echo sounds real.) Whether you're a serious scholar of folk superstitions or a bleary-eyed roulette fiend, this museum will teach you one thing: Never buy bees on a Friday.

Million-Dollar Horseshoe: at Binion's Horseshoe Casino, 128 East Fremont Street. The horseshoe is on the ground floor at the entrance nearest the corner of East Ogden Avenue and North Casino Center Boulevard. Open daily, 24 hours. Admission: free. Phone: (702) 382-1600. No one under 21 is allowed in the casino.

Ever seen a million dollars? A cool million, American cash dollars, right in front of you? Here at Binion's, in a horseshoe-shaped, five-foot-high frame are 100 $10,000 bills, neatly arranged. It's enough to make even the most staid Communist start salivating heavily. Have you ever wondered whose picture graces the $10,000 bill? Thurston Howell III's? Elvis Presley's? God's? No, it's a bland-looking politician named Salmon Portland Chase, of Chase-Manhattan Bank fame. Strangely, the backs of the bills look like play money.

Olde-Tyme Gambling Museum: in the Stardust Casino, 3000 South Las Vegas Boulevard, on the ground floor. Open daily, 10 A.M.–5:40 P.M. Admission: $1; children under 12, 50¢. Phone: (702) 732-6583.

This is alleged to be the world's largest collection of antique gambling devices, and we're not going to argue with that. Highlights include a huge collection of casino tokens and poker chips, an interesting display of cardboard lotto-type games from the 1930s and 1940s (in one game, Pork Farm, you actually win a ham), old "love-meter" machines, peep shows, horoscope machines, and more one-armed bandits than the Iraqi prison system. In another room, you learn the origin of playing cards. Life-size dioramas show what gambling halls were like in days of yore, and gambling expressions such as "dead man's hand" are explored and explained.

Ripley's Believe It or Not!: in the Four Queens Casino, 202 East Fremont Street (at Casino Center Boulevard), main floor. Open Sunday–Thursday, 9 A.M.–midnight; Friday–Saturday, 9 A.M.–1 A.M. Admission: $4.95; seniors, $3.95; children 12 and under, $2.50. Phone: (702) 385-4011. In theory, no one under 21 is allowed in the casino, but if you're going directly to Ripley's, they'll let you bring children with you.

This book is, as the cover says, a guide to unusual sights. By "unusual," we mean strange, funny, macabre, bizarre, wacky, or weird. This is not a guidebook to merely obscure or unknown places. Although many bizarre places are little known, a few of the wackiest places happen to be well known and heavily advertised. Still, their fame makes them no less strange. So if Ripley's Believe It or Not! is full of curiosities described in Robert Ripley's columns—natural anomalies, ethnic eccentricities, torture scenes, and wax figures of remarkable weirdos— we're not going to feel guilty about including it in the book. We're going to say, "Two tickets, please." The Las Vegas Ripley's has about ten different theme areas, with a special section devoted, appropriately enough, to gambling.

Tropical Laser Light Show: in the swimming pool area of the Tropicana Hotel, 3801 Las Vegas Boulevard (at Tropicana Avenue). Three shows nightly: 8:45, 10, and 11 P.M. Admission: free. Phone: (702) 739-2222.

"How dare you wake the greatest rock god since Jerry Lee Lewis?" intones the Tiki God, a laser-animated face quivering against a waterfall. Laser-generated tropical fish, boats, and other Polynesiana cavort around the lagoon, as voices with island accents—a shameless blend of Jamaica, Hawaii, and Manhattan—bounce off the shimmering rocks. This luau-for-the-eyes climaxes with a burst of color: dancing waters and a laser-fireworks extravaganza.

PANACA
(160 miles northeast of Las Vegas)

Cathedral Gorge: two miles north of Panaca; entry road branches to the west from Highway 93. Always open. Trails lead to the various sights. Phone: (702) 728-4467.

Nevada has some weird landscapes, and this is one of the weirdest. A four-mile trail takes you past formations so peculiar you'll be glad you never attempted to study geology. Some areas look like armies of alien mud monsters descending from the hills. Other areas have striated columns that seem to be emerging from the ground rather than disintegrating into it, which is what they're supposed to be doing. The geologists' attempts to explain it all only made us more disoriented. Are you sure we're still on earth?

RENO

Eddie's Fabulous '50s Casino and Diner: 45 West 2nd Street. Open daily, 24 hours. Admission: free. Phone: (800)426-6220 or (702)329-1950.

The employees wear cheerleading uniforms, letter sweaters, and saddle oxfords. Every 52 minutes, they strike a pose and do the stroll. The coffee shop is not a coffee shop but a diner, where a soda jerk keeps the beat and the cash register sits on a '57 Chevy. At the Drive-In Bar, customers huddle in old cars (which are cut in half for easy access) and watch black-and-white '50s flicks on the wide screen, while gum-popping waitresses dole out the drinks, drive-in style. Copasetic casino, Daddy-O.

Jungle in the Library: Reno Central Branch, 301 South Center Street (at Liberty Street). Open Monday–Wednesday, 10 A.M.–8:50 P.M.; Thursday–Friday, noon–5:50 P.M.; Saturday, 1–4:50 P.M. Closed Sunday. Phone: (702) 785-4190.

If Tarzan could read, you'd find him here. Over 1,300 growing plants flourish in this library—from 25-foot trees

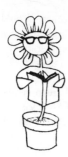

to corn to ferns to philodendrons. Landscape artists, designing the new library 20 years ago, thought plants would be a novel motif. When the library opened and patrons saw all the plants, they started donating some of their own. The library became sort of a vegetable adoption center. Humidifiers and Gro-Lite tubes make life pleasant for the plants, who are probably thanking their own plant gods that they ended up here and not in some downtown casino.

Lucky Forest: in Fitzgerald's Casino, 255 North Virginia (at Commercial), second floor. Open daily, 9 A.M.–10 P.M. Admission: free. Phone: (702) 785-3300. No one under 21 is allowed in the casino.

This Lucky Forest is a lot like the one in Las Vegas (which see). It explores good luck, bad luck, and gambling superstitions, and there's an Irish background theme, including some more Blarney stones and some antique slot machines thrown in for good measure.

Reno-Tahoe Gaming Academy: Meet tour guide at the Visitors' Center Building, 135 North Sierra Street. Tours depart Monday–Friday at 12:30 and 2 P.M. Admission: $5. Phone: (702) 348-7788.

You say you never got a chance to study gambling in college? The Gaming Academy, set up to resemble a real casino, has blackjack tables, roulette wheels, and trained gambling instructors who actually teach you how to bet, how to reckon odds, and even how to deal. While "studying" you get to play—with the Academy's money, not your own. The tour moves on to a behind-the-scenes security catwalk at a real casino, from which you can watch people gambling with their own money. Your tour guide tells of big winners, big losers, and big cheaters. (Don't miss the academy's huge collection of crooked dice.)

Wilbur D. May Museum: in Rancho San Rafael Regional Park, 1502 Washington Street, north of downtown. Open June–September, Tuesday–Sunday, 10 A.M.–5 P.M.; October–May, Wednesday–Sunday, 10 A.M.–5 P.M. Admission: $2; children, $1. Phone: (702) 785-5961.

Wilbur May went around the world 40 times. Would you expect anything different from a department store heir, pilot, big-game slaughterer, and composer of the postflapper classic "Pass a Piece of Pizza, Please"? The museum houses May's collection of souvenirs, enough to fill the world's largest curio shop: musical instruments, jewelry, eccentric antiques, photos of safaris....Visitors may even touch fur samples from exotic, if deceased, animals.

RHYOLITE
(Four miles west of Beatty)

Rhyolite Bottle House: You can't miss it among the ruins of the ghost town of Rhyolite. To get there, go west from Beatty three miles on Highway 374, then up a side road branching to the right for one mile. Always open. Admission: free. For more information, call the Beatty Chamber of Commerce at (702) 553-2721.

Rhyolite's history of eccentricity goes back to the dawn of the century, when one of the residents decided to build his house out of bottles. People laughed at him then, but he's laughing now, up in that great ghost town in the sky, as his bottle house was so well built that it's one of the few buildings left standing in the whole town. The little house is closed, but you can peer through the windows and poke around in the junk-strewn yard. The bottles, held together with cement, have been colored a faint purple by the sun's rays.

SPARKS

The Elvis Collection: inside the Sierra 76 truck stop, 200 North McCarran Boulevard, in the eastern part of town. (Take exit 19 off Interstate 80.) Open daily, 24 hours. Admission: free. Phone: (702) 359-0550.

Maybe we're revealing a secret here, but The Elvis Collection used to go by the more virile title, "Guns of Elvis." (Kind of trips off the tongue, doesn't it?) As the glass case slowly revolves, it plays Elvis' music. Inside, you'll see his photos, gargantuan jewelry, and—yup—guns, including one that the King smuggled into the United States while serving in the army. All of these items were gifts from Elvis to his father. What's it doing here? The truck stop owner met, while traveling, Vernon

Presley's girlfriend. She also happened to be the executrix of the old man's will. *Aha.*

TONOPAH

Lunar Crater Volcanic Field: 80 miles east of Tonopah, south of Highway 6, east of Sandy Summit. Visible anytime. Bring your own water, as none is available at the site. Admission: free. For more information, call (702) 482-6214.

It really does look like the surface of the moon—or like a huge bomb went off in the middle of the desert. Millions of years of volcanic activity along a fault line produced over 100 eerie square miles of lava flows, cinder cones, and yawning craters. Lunar Crater, once a mighty volcano, measures nearly a mile across and is 430 feet deep. Four miles southeast on Highway 6 is Easy Chair Crater, named for its resemblance to a living-room chair. It was formed when the side of a volcano—instead of the top—blew off.

VIRGINIA CITY

Camel and Ostrich Races: the Friday, Saturday, and Sunday after Labor Day, usually around September 10. Races on Friday are at 7 P.M., at the V & T Railroad depot. Races on Saturday and Sunday run all day, following the 11 A.M. camel and ostrich parade on C Street; races are at the Amphitheatre on F Street. Admission: $6 (gets you in for all races on all three days). Phone: (702) 883-7223.

What started in 1959 as a phony news story has blossomed into one of the state's wackiest annual events. In 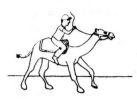1960, the journalistic practical joke turned into reality when three camels showed up, ready to race, jockeys in tow. Oddly, the first victorious jockey was director John Huston. Two years later, ostriches joined the bill, and now Virginia City is a world center for camel and ostrich racing. Camels, unlike horses, don't like to do what humans tell them. That goes double for ostriches, especially when they're forced to drag little chariots behind them. Expect havoc.

Gambling Museum: inside the Palace Emporium Mall, downtown. Museum is located behind 20 South C Street, across the street from the Delta parking lot. Open daily, 10 A.M.–5 P.M. Admission: $1.50; children under 12, free. Phone: (702) 847-0787.

From Native American knucklebone games to bloody bull and bear fights, this museum traces the history of Nevada's favorite sport. Many of the slot machines here have glass fronts: You can play them and get a close look at their digestive processes. Also of interest is a replica of a 19th-century saloon and a taxidermed bobcat—a souvenir of Virginia City's fleeting flirtation with dog and cat fights.

The Silver Queen: on the wall at the Silver Queen Casino, 9 North C Street. Look to your right as you enter the casino. Open daily, 10 A.M.–10 P.M. Admission: free. Phone: (702) 847-0440.

This 16-foot-tall painted lady looks more like a dancehall amazon than a queen. She's got a high price on her; that's for sure. Silver dollars form the fabric of her gown: 3,261 of them, in all. Twenty-eight $20 gold pieces form her belt, and three rows of silver dollars march all around the perimeter. The Queen was created in memory of Virginia City's silver-mining salad days.

Territorial Prison: 70 South C Street (at Washington). Open daily, 10 A.M.–5 P.M. Admission: 50¢; children under 6, free. Phone: (702) 847-0500. Ask for Earl or Anne-Marie.

A prison marshall takes your four bits and lets you in to see the sorry inmates of the Territorial Prison. Oops—the executioner's taking his coffee break; you can do his job for him by dropping a dime in the slot and zapping the remorseless prisoner in the electric chair. Sad-faced criminals do their time in the cells, ignoring yet another execution victim who swings from a rope. Did we forget to mention that these are all dummies, not real people? Sorry about that.

WEST WENDOVER

Unique Viewpoint: follow Wendover's Main Street (which is *not* the highway) west from the Nevada-Utah border through West Wendover, up the hill until you come to a dirt turnaround. The view is toward the east. For more information, call (702) 664-3414.

Because of this mountain's position overlooking Utah's legendary Bonneville Salt Flats, it is the only place on land where you can clearly see the curvature of the earth. The Salt Flats are as flat as flat can be, stretching off to the horizon. Locals say the best time to visit is at dusk, when "it looks like you're on the edge of the world."

BASQUE FESTIVALS

Northern Spain and southwestern France are the ancestral home of the Basques, a mysterious, culturally proud people whose language is like no other on earth and who brought the world black wool berets and the game of jai alai. Great numbers of Basques, fleeing war and poverty at home, arrived in Nevada 100 years ago, found work in the sheepherding trade, and are today one of the state's most visible ethnic groups. Several cities hold annual Basque festivals, at which you can watch traditional Basque contests and belly up to the traditionally vast servings of beans, lamb, and sheepherders' bread. Don't miss a chance to see *irrintzi*, a Basque yelling competition.

Here are some of Nevada's Basque festivals:
Elko: July 4 weekend. Elko County Fairgrounds, Elko City Park (on Idaho Street) and the Elko Convention Center (Festival Way). Some events have an admission fee. Phone: (702) 738-7135 or (702) 738-3295.

Thousands flock to Nevada's biggest—and oldest—Basque gathering to enjoy wood chopping, weight lifting, bread baking, and *irrintzi* contests. There's also a tug-of-war, hoop and wineglass dances, and a Catholic mass held in the Basque language.
Ely: third Saturday in July. Broadbent Park, on Highway 6. Admission to barbecue: $10. Phone: (702) 289-2100.

Whole lambs are barbecued on a spit. The feast also includes sausage, salad, beans, and wine. Collies demonstrate their sheepherding skills; men compete at weight carrying and wood chopping.

Las Vegas: first or second weekend in September (varies). Silk Purse Ranch, Tonopah Highway at Durango Drive, northwest Las Vegas. Indoor events take place at St. Viator Community Center, Flamingo Road at Eastern Avenue. Admission: $2. Phone: (702) 361-6834.

Wood-chopping contests—a Basque favorite and a test of both speed and strength—are a highlight here. Other contests as well as edibles enhance the fun.

Reno: the last Saturday in August, 10 A.M.–1 A.M. Nevada State Fairgrounds, just off Interstate 80 at the Wells turnoff. Admission: $12; children, $6. Phone: (800) 367-7366.

Go, dog, go! Sheepdog races, weightlifting contests, team tug-of-war, and past-midnight dancing make up Reno's Basque event.

Winnemucca: Fathers' Day weekend. Humboldt County Fairgrounds, eastern end of town. Admission: $2. Phone: (702) 623-3192 or (702) 623-5071.

Competitors carry two 100-pound weights (one in each hand) a distance of 100 feet. Other activities include sheepdog exhibitions, a Basque mass, a picnic, and folk dances.

EPILOGUE

THE ONES THAT GOT AWAY

While traveling around and researching this book, we discovered to our dismay that some of the most remarkable off-the-wall sites we had been searching for were out of business, were bulldozed, had closed up, had moved, or had simply vanished without a trace. You may be wondering why we neglected to mention in this guide a certain wacky amusement park you once visited years ago or a bizarre museum about which you've heard wild rumors. In most cases, sadly, there is no longer an amusement park or museum left to visit. So in case you think we've been derelict in our duties as connoisseurs of the weird, here's a selective compendium of the ones that got away, the legendary and mysterious attractions that are now—sniff— only a memory.

Fresno's Forestiere Underground Gardens is closed because of legal entanglements; the Frisbee Museum of Las Vegas has moved to points unknown; The Magicians' Hall of Fame in Hollywood seems never to be open; Wonder Hill in Salinas lost its mystical properties when a freeway was built next door; The Dalles' Bigfoot Museum disappeared into the woods; the Stanford Apports and Occult Collection are not on display to the public; Nellie Bly O'Bryan's Upside-Down House at Mono Lake is now just a crumbling shack; the miraculous Face of Jesus Stove of Oroville is lost and unaccounted for; Seattle's Western Union Museum is permanently closed; very little remains of The Ministry of Universal Wisdom's Giant Rock Airport near Yucca Valley; Loboland has moved from Port Angeles to a different part of the country; Wilbur Bradley's Gourd Farm in National City is gone; The Crypotozoology Museum in Los Angeles has yet to open; San Francisco's Emperor

Herbal Restaurant is out of business; Possom Trot in Yermo has been destroyed; The Alligator Farm in Buena Park is gone; Shady Cove's Uncanny Canyon is now at the bottom of a reservoir; The Museum of the Ordinary in Sausalito was dismantled; The Devil's Inkwell at The Geysers is now underneath a geothermal power plant; Eaglemont Rockeries of Port Townsend is no longer open to the public; the desert religious statues of Rhyolite are gone; Los Angeles' Weird Museum burned down; Lost World north of Santa Cruz was closed, though the Tree Circus was moved to Gilroy; Cecil B. DeMille's cinematic Egyptian ruins in the Guadalupe Dunes are closed to the public; the Grants Pass Garlic Festival was cancelled; the University of California at San Francisco Anatomy Museum is not on exhibit; Athena's Jaws of Mystery Museum is gone; San Francisco's Rock and Roll museum has not yet found a home; the Ben Franklin Museum of Portland was dismantled; Santa's Village north of Santa Cruz went out of business; the Tropico World Gold Panning Championship moved to another part of the country; and San Francisco's Museum of Package Antiquities is in storage, waiting for a new location.

Let it also be noted that we purposely excluded, with only a couple of exceptions, all doll museums and car museums, as there are far too many of them and they rarely pass our strict "off-the-wall" criteria. And one final mournful tale: We spent a great deal of time and energy tracking down ghost towns, only to find that almost every one had been destroyed by vandals, treasure hunters, wind, rain, and encroaching suburbia. Like the buffalo, they were once common but have now been driven almost to extinction. Treat the few ghost towns listed here as you would the last members of an endangered species.

GENERAL INDEX

SPECIAL INDEXES

BUILDINGS SHAPED LIKE THINGS

ECCENTRIC ART

Piercy, CA, Confusion Hill, 134
Rohnert Park, CA, Gravity Anomaly, 137
Santa Cruz, CA, The Mystery Spot, 60

RENAISSANCE AND MEDIEVAL FAIRES

Agoura Hills, CA, Renaissance Pleasure Faire, 22
Carnation, WA, Camlann Medieval Faire, 176
Grants Pass, OR, Renaissance Fair, 154
Hanford, CA, Renaissance of Kings Fair, 72
Novato, CA, Renaissance Pleasure Faire, 96
Richland, WA, Ye Merrie Greenwood Faire, 189
San Luis Obispo, CA, Renaissance Faire, 58
Sherwood, OR, Robin Hood Festival, 170
Walla Walla, WA, Renaissance Faire, 201

SAND CASTLE CONTESTS

Alameda, CA, 88
Bandon, OR, 144
Birch Bay, WA, 175
Cannon Beach, OR, 148
Capitola, CA, 50
Carmel, CA, 50
Copalis Beach, WA, 177
Lincoln City, OR, 160
Long Beach, CA, 34
Long Beach, WA, 183
Manhattan Beach, CA, 38
Newport Beach, CA, 40
Pismo Beach, CA, 56
Port Orford, OR, 167
Rockaway, OR, 168
San Diego, CA, 18
Santa Barbara, CA, 59
Seattle, WA, 195
Waldport, OR, 172

SLUG FESTIVALS

Eatonville, WA, Slug Festival, 178
Elma, WA, The Elma Slug Festival, 179
Fairhaven, WA, Slug Race, 179
Florence, OR, Slug Race, 152
Kingston, WA, Slug Race, 181
Monte Rio, CA, Slug Festival, 130
Orick, CA, Slug Derby, 131
Santa Cruz, CA, UCSC Slug Fest, 61
Waldport, OR, Beachcomber Days, 172